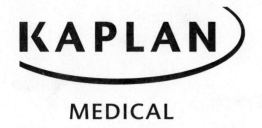

MEDICAL

USMLE®

STEP 2 CK

**Lecture Notes
2016**

**Psychiatry,
Epidemiology,
Ethics,
Patient Safety**

© 2015 by Kaplan, Inc.

Published by Kaplan Medical, a division of Kaplan, Inc.
750 Third Avenue
New York, NY 10017

Printed in the United States of America
10 9 8 7 6 5 4 3 2 1

Course ISBN: 978-1-62523-669-2 | Item Number: BL4021L

Retail Kit ISBN: 978-1-5062-0087-3
This item comes as a set and should not be broken out and sold separately.

Kaplan Publishing print books are available at special quantity discounts to use for sales promotions, employee premiums, or educational purposes. For more information or topurchase books, please call the Simon & Schuster special sales department at 866-506-1949.

EDITORS

Psychiatry
Alina Gonzalez-Mayo, M.D.
Psychiatrist
Dept. of Veteran's Administration
Bay Pines, FL

Patient Safety and Quality Improvement
Ted A. James, M.D., M.S., F.A.C.S.
Medical Director, Clinical Simulation and Patient Safety
Director, Skin & Soft Tissue Surgical Oncology
Associate Professor of Surgery
University of Vermont College of Medicine
Burlington, VT

Contents

Psychiatry

Epidemiology & Ethics

Patient Safety and Quality Improvement

Index

Psychiatry

Mental Status Examination

The mental status examination is used to describe the clinician's observations and impressions of the patient during the interview. In conjunction with the history of the patient, it is the best way to make an accurate diagnosis.

General Description

- *Appearance:* grooming, poise, clothes, body type (disheveled, neat, childlike, etc.)
- *Behavior:* quantitative and qualitative aspects of the patient's motor behavior (restless, tics, etc.)
- *Attitude toward the examiner:* (cooperative, frank, and seductive)

Mood and Affect

- *Mood:* emotions perceived by the patient (depressed, anxious, angry, etc.)
- *Affect:* patient's present emotional responsiveness (blunted, flat, labile, etc.)
- *Appropriateness:* in reference to the context of the subject (appropriate or inappropriate)

Speech: The physical characteristics of speech (relevant, coherent, fluent, etc.)

Perceptual disturbances: Experienced in reference to self or the environment (hallucinations, illusions)

- *Hallucinations:* false sensory perceptions without a stimulus
    - Auditory: psychotic disorders
    - Visual: drugs, organic diseases
    - Tactile: cocaine intoxication, alcohol withdrawal
    - Olfactory: seizures
- *Illusions:* sensory misperception with a stimulus

Thought

- *Form of thought:* the way in which a person thinks (flight of ideas, loose associations, tangentiality, circumstantiality, etc.)
- *Content of thought:* what the person is actually thinking about (delusions, paranoia, and suicidal ideas)

Sensorium and Cognition

- Alertness and level of consciousness (awake, clouding of consciousness, etc.)
- Orientation: time, place, and person
- Memory: recent, remote, recent past, and immediate retention and recall
- Concentration and attention: serial sevens, ability to spell backwards.
- Capacity to read and write: Ask patient to read a sentence and perform what it says.

- Visuospatial ability: copy a figure
- Abstract thinking: similarities and proverb interpretation
- Fund of information and knowledge: calculating ability, name past presidents

Impulse Control: Estimated from history or behavior during the interview

Judgment and Insight: Ability to act appropriately and self-reflect

Reliability: Physician's impressions of the patient's ability to accurately assess his situation

Interviewing Techniques

Open-Ended Questions: Allow the patient to speak in his own words as much as possible.

> "Can you describe your pain?"

Closed-Ended Questions: Ask for specific information without allowing options in answering.

> "Are you hearing voices?"

Facilitation: Physician helps the patient continue by providing verbal and nonverbal cues.

> "Yes, please continue."

Confrontation: Physician points something out to the patient.

> "You seem very upset today."

Leading: The answer in the question.

> "Are the voices telling you to hurt yourself?"

Review Questions

1. A 20-year-old man presents to your office complaining of auditory hallucinations for approximately 7 months in duration. He reports hearing his father's voice and at times his mother's voice as well. The patient appears distressed by the hallucinations and wants your help. Which of the following would be the most appropriate statement at this time?

   (A) "What do the voices say?"
   (B) "Have you taken medication?"
   (C) "Why do you think you hear voices?"
   (D) "How is your relationship with your parents?"
   (E) "Tell me about the voices."

2. A 30-year-old woman comes to see you after her mother's death approximately 3 weeks ago. Since then she has complained of depressed mood and feelings of helplessness. While in your office, she begins to cry. Which of the following would be the next step in the management of this patient?

   (A) Say, "I will come back when you stop crying."
   (B) Say, "Do you feel guilty about your mother's death?"
   (C) Offer tissue and remain silent
   (D) Say, "Go ahead; it is normal to cry."
   (E) Refer to a psychiatrist for further evaluation

1. **Answer: E.** The ideal interviewing technique is to begin with an open-ended question and conclude with closed-ended questions. Choices A, C, D, and E are all open-ended questions. However, the best open-ended question for this patient and the reason he came to see you is choice E.

2. **Answer: C.** One should always express empathy and then give the patient control. By staying silent and offering a tissue, you are doing just that. Choice E is always incorrect.

Defense Mechanisms 2

Id: Drives (instincts) present at birth. The 2 most important drives are sex and aggression.

Ego: Defense mechanisms, judgment, relationship to reality, object relationships, developed shortly after birth

Superego: Conscience, empathy, and morality are formed during latency period, right vs. wrong

DEFENSE MECHANISMS

Defense mechanisms are the way and means that the **ego** wards off anxiety and controls instinctive urges and unpleasant emotions. They are unconscious (except suppression), discrete, dynamic and irreversible, and may be adaptive or maladaptive.

Types of Defense Mechanisms

Projection: Attributing your own wishes, thoughts, or feelings onto someone else.

> "I'm sure my wife is cheating on me."

Denial: Used to avoid becoming aware of some painful aspect of reality.

> "I know I do not have cancer."

Splitting: External objects are divided into all good or all bad.

> "The morning staff is perfect, the evening staff is terrible."

Blocking: Temporary block in thinking.

> "I have known him for years but can never seem to remember his name."

Regression: Return to an earlier stage of development, most immature.

> "Ever since my divorce, my 5-year-old has begun to wet the bed."

Somatization: Psychic derivatives are converted into bodily symptoms.

> "Just thinking of the exam I get butterflies in my stomach."

Introjection: Features of the external world are taken and made part of the self.

> The resident physician dresses like the attending whom he admires.

Displacement: An emotion or drive is shifted to another that resembles the original in some aspect.

> "I had to get rid of the dog since my husband kicked it every time we had an argument."

Repression: An idea or feeling is withheld from consciousness; unconscious forgetting.

> "I do not remember having had a dog."

Intellectualization: Excessive use of intellectual processes to avoid affective expression or experience.

> "It is interesting to note the specific skin lesions which seem to arise as a consequence of my end-stage disease."

Isolation: Separation of an idea from the affect that accompanies it.

> "As she arrived at the station to identify the body, she appeared to show no emotion."

Rationalization: Rational explanations are used to justify unacceptable attitudes, beliefs, or behaviors.

> "I did not pass the test because it was harder this year than ever before."

Reaction formation: An unacceptable impulse is transformed into its opposite; results in the formation of character traits.

> "Listen to him tell his family he was not afraid, when I saw him crying."

Undoing: Acting out the reverse of an unacceptable behavior; consists of an act.

> "I need to wash my hands whenever I have these thoughts."

Acting out: Behavioral or emotional outburst.

> "My 10-year-old started getting into trouble right after his mother and I got divorced."

Humor: Permits the expression of feelings and thoughts without personal discomfort.

> "So," said the 300-pound man, "they expected me to place my head between my legs in the event of a plane crash when the best I could manage was placing my chin on my chest."

Sublimation: Impulse gratification has been achieved, but the aim or object has been changed from unacceptable to acceptable; allows instincts to be channeled. Most mature of the defenses.

> Jack the Ripper becomes a surgeon.

Suppression: Conscious forgetting; only conscious defense mechanism.

> "I would rather talk about my operation after the party is over."

Dissociation: Splitting off of the brain from conscious awareness.

> "I hardly remember getting to the hospital after my husband was hit by a car."

Review Question

A nurse, working in a hospice, has been ignoring an elderly female patient who has terminal cancer. When asked why she has been ignoring the patient, the nurse replied, "She wants to be left alone." Which of the following defense mechanisms best explains her response?

(A)   Rationalization
(B)   Isolation of affect
(C)   Intellectualization
(D)   Projection
(E)   Denial

Answer: D. The nurse is projecting her wishes by stating that the patient wants to be left alone, when in reality it is *she* who wants to be left alone. Rationalization (A) is making excuses for your behavior. Had that been the answer, she would have made excuses, such as she's too busy, etc.

TESTS

Intelligence Tests

Intelligence Quotient (IQ) measures academic performance.

$$IQ = MA/CA \times 100; \text{ Mean IQ} = 100 \text{ (SD} = 15)$$

Adults: Wechsler Adult Intelligence Scale Revised (WAIS-R)

Children: Wechsler Intelligence Scale for Children Revised (WISC-R), Stanford-Binet

Personality Tests

Objective tests use simple stimuli, do not need much clinical experience: Minnesota Multiphasic Personality Inventory (MMPI).

Projective tests use ambiguous stimuli, need clinical experience, not diagnostic: Rorschach test (inkblot), Thematic Apperception Test (TAT), sentence completion tests, family drawings.

Childhood Disorders 3

INTELLECTUAL DISABILITY (ID)

Definition. Formerly called mental retardation. Significantly subaverage intellectual function (IQ <70), as measured by a variety of IQ tests. This must be accompanied by concurrent impairment in adapting to demands of school, work, social, and other environments. Onset is age <18.

Risk Factors/Etiology. Associated genetic and chromosomal abnormalities include inborn errors of metabolism (e.g., lipidoses, aminoacidurias, glycogen storage diseases) and chromosomal abnormalities (e.g., cri du chat syndrome, Down syndrome, fragile X syndrome). Associated intrauterine infections include rubella, cytomegalovirus, and other viruses. Intrauterine exposure to toxins and other insults such as alcohol, hypoxia, or malnutrition may be causal. Postnatal causes include exposure to toxins and infection, poor prenatal care, postnatal exposure to heavy metals, physical trauma, and social deprivation.

Presenting Symptoms

- *Prevalence:* 1% of the population. Occurs at a 1.2:1 male-to-female ratio.

- *Mild ID (IQ 50–69):* Attain academic skills to approximately the sixth-grade level, often live independently in the community or with minimal supervision, may have problems with impulse control and self-esteem, and may have associated conduct disorders, substance-related disorders, and attention deficit hyperactivity disorder (ADHD).

- *Moderate ID (IQ 35–50):* Attain academic skills to a second-grade level, may be able to manage activities of daily living, work in sheltered workshops, live in residential community settings, and have significant problems conforming to social norms. Individuals with Down's syndrome are at high risk for early development of Alzheimer's disease.

- *Severe (IQ 20–35) and profound ID (IQ <20):* Little or no speech, very limited abilities to manage self-care, requires highly supervised care settings.

Physical Examination. Evidence of underlying disorder or injury

Diagnostic Tests. Amniocentesis: May reveal chromosomal abnormalities associated with ID in high-risk pregnancies (mother age >35.)

Treatment. Primary prevention includes genetic counseling, good prenatal care, and safe environments. Treatment of associated general medical conditions may improve overall level of cognitive and adaptive function. Special education techniques may improve ultimate level of function. Behavioral guidance and attention to promoting self-esteem may improve long-term emotional adjustment.

Differential Diagnosis. Includes learning and communication disorders, sensory impairment, autism spectrum disorder, borderline intellectual functioning (IQ 70–100), and environmental deprivation.

LEARNING DISORDERS

Definition. Characterized by learning achievement in specific areas that is substantially below expectations, given the patient's age, intelligence, sensory abilities, and educational experience. Types of learning disorder are reading disorder (most common), mathematics disorder, and disorder of written expression.

Risk Factors/Etiology. Some cases are due to the effects of coexisting general medical conditions such as cerebral palsy on central nervous system (CNS) function. Some general medical conditions and substance-induced conditions are associated with learning disorders, including lead poisoning and fetal alcohol syndrome. Many cases have no obvious etiology.

Presenting Symptoms

- Prevalence: 5% of school-age children
- Onset: usually during elementary school
- Perceptual–motor problems
- Conduct disorder, oppositional defiant disorder, and ADHD
- Poor self-esteem and social immaturity
- School failure and behavioral disturbances

Deficits sometimes persist into adulthood and interfere with occupational function.

Diagnostic Tests. IQ testing and academic achievement tests are the major diagnostic tools.

Treatment. Special education to ensure general learning and maximize skills in the deficient areas is the mainstay of treatment. Counseling of patients and families to improve self-esteem, social behavior, and family functioning is helpful.

Differential Diagnosis. Major rule-outs are environmental deprivation, hearing or vision impairment, and ID.

AUTISM SPECTRUM DISORDERS (ASD)

Definition: A group of disorders characterized by problems with social interaction, behavior, and language.

Risk Factors/Etiology. The cause is CNS damage due to known or unknown factors. Sites of CNS damage specifically associated with ASD are unknown. General medical conditions associated with ASD include encephalitis, maternal rubella, PKU, tuberous sclerosis, fragile X syndrome, and perinatal anoxia. There is no obvious etiology in many cases.

Presenting Symptoms

- *Prevalence:* 0.08% of the general population. Occurs at a 5:1 male-to-female ratio.
- *Onset:* Before 3 years of age
- *Social symptoms:* Lack of peer relationships and a failure to use nonverbal social cues
- *Communication symptoms:* Absent or bizarre use of speech
- *Behavioral symptoms:* Odd preoccupation with repetitive activities, bizarre mannerisms, and rigid adherence to purposeless ritual
- ID is present in 75% of patients with ASD.
- *Physical findings:* Higher incidence of abnormal electroencephalograms (EEGs), seizures, and abnormal brain morphology

- *Course:* Approximately 30% of individuals with ASD become semi-independent in adulthood, but almost all have severe residual disabilities.
- Predictors of a poor outcome are associated ID and failure to develop useful speech.
- Seizures develop by adulthood in 25% of autistic individuals.

Physical Examination. Self-injuries caused by head banging or biting sometimes present.

Treatment. The major treatment is family counseling, special education, and newer antipsychotic medications to control episodes of severe agitation or self-destructive behavior.

Differential Diagnosis. Major rule-outs are ID, hearing impairment, environmental deprivation, selective mutism, and Rett syndrome.

ATTENTION DEFICIT HYPERACTIVITY DISORDER (ADHD)

Definition. ADHD is characterized by inattention, hyperactivity, and impulsivity that interfere with social or academic function. Symptoms last for at least 6 months, and onset occurs before age 12. Symptoms are present in multiple settings. Subtypes are based on the predominance of symptoms of inattention or of hyperactivity and impulsivity.

Risk Factors/Etiology. No specific etiologies have been identified. Other CNS pathology and disadvantaged family and school situations are sometimes present.

Prevalence. 5% of school-age children and 2.5% of adults. Male-to-female ratio is 2:1 in children and 1.6:1 in adults.

Family history. ADHD, mood and anxiety disorders, substance-related disorders, and antisocial personality disorder.

Onset. Usually first recognized when a child enters school, and symptoms usually persist throughout childhood. ADHD, particularly the attention deficit, persists into adulthood in most but not all affected individuals. Hyperactivity tends to diminish in adolescence and adulthood.

Symptoms. Short attention span, constant fidgeting, inability to sit through cartoons or meals, inability to wait in lines, failure to stay quiet or sit still in class, disobedience, shunning by peers, fighting, poor academic performance, carelessness, and poor relationships with siblings.

Common Associated Problems. Low self-esteem, mood lability, conduct disorder, learning disorders, clumsiness, communication disorders, drug abuse, school failure, and physical trauma as a result of impulsivity.

Physical Examination. Perceptual: motor problems and poor coordination may be present.

Diagnostic Tests. IQ tests and various structured symptom-rating scales for use by teachers and parents are often used.

Differential Diagnosis. Major rule-outs are age-appropriate behavior, response to environmental problems, ID, ASD, and mood disorders.

Treatment. Target symptoms are defined before initiating treatment. Psychological, social, and educational interventions include adding structure and stability to home and school environments. Specialized educational techniques include the use of multiple sensory modalities for teaching, instructions that are short and frequently repeated, immediate reinforcement for learning, and minimization of classroom distractions. Pharmacotherapy of choice is stimulant medications, such as methylphenidate and dextroamphetamine. Non-stimulants such as atomoxetine may also be used. They are usually effective in decreasing hyperactivity, inattention, and impulsivity. Other medications include antidepressants and clonidine.

CONDUCT DISORDER

Definition. Persistent violations over at least 6 months in 4 areas: aggression, property destruction, deceitfulness or theft, and rules.

Risk Factors/Etiology. Genetic influences play a role by affecting temperament. Stressful family and school environments have also been implicated.

Prevalence. 4% of school-age children. Seen more in males.

Family History. Antisocial personality disorder, conduct disorder, ADHD, mood disorders, and substance-related disorders.

Onset. Most often during late childhood or early adolescence.

Course. In most individuals, the symptoms gradually remit.

Key Symptoms. Bullying, fighting, cruelty to people or animals, and rape, vandalism, firesetting, theft, robbery, running away, school truancy

Complications. Substance-related disorders and school failures

Outcome. Often, antisocial personality disorder, somatic symptom disorders, depressive disorders, and substance-related disorders

Differential Diagnosis. Major rule-outs are environmental problems, ADHD, and oppositional defiant disorder.

Treatment. Healthy group identity and role models are provided by structured sports programs and other programs (e.g., Big Brothers). Structured living settings that place value on group identification and cooperation are useful. Punishment and incarceration are not often effective.

OPPOSITIONAL DEFIANT DISORDER

Definition. Persistent pattern lasting at least 6 months of negativistic, hostile, and defiant behaviors toward adults, including arguments, temper outbursts, vindictiveness, and deliberate annoyance.

Risk Factors/Etiology. High reactivity and increased motor behavior are innate features of temperament that may predispose to this disorder. Inconsistent or poor parenting may also contribute.

Prevalence. 3% of school-age children. Male-to-female ratio is 1:1 after puberty but boys > girls before puberty.

Onset. Usually in latency or early adolescence and may start gradually. Onset later in girls.

Associated Problems. Family conflict and school failure, low self-esteem and mood lability, early onset of substance abuse, ADHD and learning disorders.

Course. Family conflict often escalates after the onset of symptoms.

Outcome. Conduct disorder may follow.

Treatment. Parents should be advised to spend time interacting with a child, to reward desired behavior and not simply punish undesired behavior, and to be consistent in statements and deeds. Alternative caregivers may be indicated in some cases.

Differential Diagnosis. Conduct disorder

CHILDHOOD ENURESIS

Definition. The disorder is characterized by repeated voiding of urine into the patient's clothes or bed in a child at least 5 years of age. It is diagnosed only if the behavior is not due to a medical condition.

Risk Factors/Etiology. Current psychologic stress, family history of enuresis, and urinary tract infections.

Prevalence. 3–5% of children aged 10. Slightly more common in boys. May occur only at night, only during daytime, or both. Often causes emotional turmoil in the child or parents.

Physical Examination. Assessment for urinary tract infection or abnormalities should occur.

Treatment. Appropriate toilet training and avoiding large amounts of fluids before bed are important, as are decreasing emotional stressors. A bell-pad apparatus is the best treatment. Pharmacotherapy includes imipramine and desmopressin (DDAVP) for short-term treatment.

CHILDHOOD ANXIETY

Definition. Normal childhood anxiety:

- *Stranger anxiety:* Fear of strangers in unfamiliar contexts that is present from age 6 months to approximately 2 years.
- *Separation anxiety:* Fear of separation from the caregiver that is present from approximately 1 to 3 years of age.

Risk Factors/Etiology. Excessively close-knit families, excessive expectations of children, and innate temperamental anxiety

Prevalence. 5% of school-age children

Key Symptoms. Prominent physical complaints such as stomachaches and malaise, unrealistic fears (e.g., monsters) and nightmares, phobias such as school phobia and fear of animals or the dark, difficulty sleeping, and self-mutilation such as scratching, nail-biting, and hair-pulling.

Physical Examination. Evidence of nail biting and scratching is sometimes present.

Treatment. Family therapy helps parents recognize and lessen childhood anxiety. Cognitive behavioral therapy is useful to decrease anxiety in older children.

Complications. Social avoidance, low self-esteem, and inhibited social development may occur.

TOURETTE DISORDER

Definition. Childhood onset of multiple motor and vocal tics

Risk Factors/Etiology. Autosomal dominant transmission may occur in some cases. There are associations between ADHD (50%) and obsessive compulsive disorder (OCD) (40%). Abnormalities in the dopaminergic and adrenergic system have been implicated.

Prevalence. 3 per 1,000. More common in males.

Onset. Average age 7 years with motor tics and vocal tics typically appearing at age 11 years

Course. Vocal and motor tics wax and wane over time.
- *Motor tics:* May present as twitching of face, trunk, or extremities or may involve complex behaviors such as pacing, spinning, or touching.
- *Vocal tics:* Usually grunts; coprolalia (cursing) occurs in about 10% of cases.

Associated Problems. ADHD and obsessive-compulsive disorder are each present in about one-third of cases. ADHD occurs before tics whereas OCD symptoms occur after the tics.

Course. Lifelong, with remissions and exacerbations

Treatment. Antipsychotic drugs, including pimozide, haloperidol, olanzapine and risperidone are treatments of choice. Clonidine and clonazepam are sometimes useful.

Review Question

A 13-year-old boy is referred by his junior high school principal for evaluation of his short attention span and inability to sit quietly in class or on the school bus. He has a quick temper at school and at home, and his peers tease him about his temper.

Which of the following is most likely to be an associated finding in this case?

(A) Affectual blunting
(B) Autistic mannerisms
(C) Conduct disturbances
(D) Grandiosity and inflated self-esteem
(E) Intellectual disability

Answer: C. The symptoms in this case are suggestive of ADHD. Conduct disturbances are a common associated finding in individuals with ADHD; drug abuse is also more common. Affect tends to be more labile, and low self-esteem is common. Although ID is seen more often in children with ADHD than in the general population, it is not a common associated finding, and this boy is at the expected grade level for his age. ASD is rarely diagnosed in individuals with ADHD.

Used with permission from Williams & Wilkins, *Board Review Series: Psychiatry*, 1997.

Depressive, Bipolar, and Related Disorders

4

MAJOR DEPRESSIVE DISORDER (MAJOR DEPRESSION)

A 70-year-old woman was recently admitted after her son informed the doctor that she had been doing very poorly over the past few months. The patient reports a 30-pound weight loss, decreased concentration, feelings of helplessness and hopelessness, decreased energy, depressed mood, and decreased sleep.

Definition. Mood disorder that presents with at least a 2-week course of symptoms that is a change from the patient's previous level of functioning. Must have depressed mood or anhedonia (inability to enjoy oneself).

Risk Factors/Epidemiology. Major depression is seen more frequently in women due to several factors, such as hormonal differences, great stress, or simply a bias in the diagnosis. The typical age of onset is 40 years. There is also a higher incidence in those who have no close interpersonal relationships or are divorced or separated. Many studies have reported abnormalities in serotonin, norepinephrine, and dopamine. Other risk factors include family history, exposure to stressors, and behavioral reasons, such as learned helplessness.

Presenting Symptoms
- Depressed mood most of the day
- Anhedonia during most of the day
- Significant weight loss (>5% of body weight)
- Insomnia
- Psychomotor agitation or retardation
- Fatigue or loss of energy nearly every day
- Feelings of worthlessness or guilt
- Diminished ability to concentrate
- Recurrent thoughts about death

Physical Examination. Usually within normal limits; however, may find evidence of psychomotor retardation, such as stooped posture, slowing of movements, slowed speech, etc. May also find evidence of cognitive impairment, such as decreased concentration and forgetfulness.

May also include:
- *Psychotic features:* Worse prognosis
- *Atypical features:* Increased weight, appetite, and sleep

Treatment. Must first secure the safety of the patient, given that suicide is such a high risk. Pharmacotherapy includes antidepressant medications such as SSRIs. Tricyclic antidepressants (TCAs), or monoamine oxidase inhibitors (MAOIs). Electroconvulsive therapy (ECT) may be indicated if patient is suicidal or intolerant to medications. Individual psychotherapy is indicated to help the patient deal with conflicts, sense of loss, etc. Another form of therapy is cognitive therapy, which will change the patient's distorted thoughts about self, future, world, etc.

Differential Diagnosis. *Medical disorders:* Hypothyroidism, Parkinson's disease, dementia, medications such as hypertensives, pseudodementia, tumors, cerebrovascular accidents. *Mental disorders:* Other mood disorders, substance disorders, and grief.

BIPOLAR I DISORDER

> A 19-year-old college student is taken to the school counselor after he fails several classes. The patient is enrolled in numerous classes, most of which have conflicting times. His grades are poor, and he seems undisturbed by this. He is also enrolled in numerous organizations, such as the chess club, drama club, student government, sports, and at least two fraternities. His speech is pressured and he has psychomotor agitation.

Definition. A mood disturbance in which the patient typically experiences symptoms of elevated mood, for at least 1 week that cause significant distress or impairment in his/her level of functioning.

Risk Factors/Epidemiology. Bipolar disorder affects men and women equally and has a mean age of onset of about 18 years. More prevalent among high socioeconomic status. Considered to be the illness with the greatest genetic linkage. Coexisting disorders may include anxiety, alcohol dependence, and substance-related disorders.

Presenting Symptoms

- Abnormal or persistently elevated mood lasting at least 1 week
- Increased self-esteem or grandiosity
- Distractibility
- Excessive involvement in activities
- More talkative than usual
- Psychomotor agitation
- Flight of ideas
- Increased sexual activity
- Increase in goal-directed activity

Physical Examination. Usually within normal limits; however, may find evidence of psychomotor agitation and pressured speech.

Treatment. Must assess patient safety to determine the need for hospitalization. Pharmacotherapy will include mood stabilizers, benzodiazepines, and antipsychotics.

Differential Diagnosis

- *Mental disorders:* Schizophrenia, personality disorders, and bipolar II disorder (includes major depressive episodes and hypomanic but not manic episodes)
- *Medical disorders:* CNS infections, tumors, hyperthyroidism, and medications

PERSISTENT DEPRESSIVE DISORDER (DYSTHYMIA)

Mr. Smith complains of poor appetite, low energy, poor concentration, and difficulty in making decisions, which affects his ability to complete his assignments at work. These symptoms have been present for more than 2 years.

Definition. A chronic disorder characterized by a depressed mood that lasts most of the time during the day and is present on most days for at least 2 years.

Risk Factors/Epidemiology. Patients typically have other psychiatric disorders, such as anxiety, substance abuse, and/or borderline personality disorders.

Treatment. Hospitalization is usually not indicated in these patients. They may benefit from psychotherapy to help them overcome their long-term sense of despair and resolve conflicts from childhood. If medications are indicated, SSRIs, TCAs, or MAOIs are usually preferred.

Differential Diagnosis. Differential diagnosis is essentially the same as for major depression.

CYCLOTHYMIC DISORDER

Mrs. McDonald has experienced a 12-year history of periods of feeling great followed by periods of feeling lousy. During her feeling-great periods, she experiences increased sexual drive, euphoric mood, and increased irritability. During her feeling-lousy periods, she experiences insomnia, fatigue, and low self-esteem.

Definition. A chronic disorder characterized by many periods of depressed mood and many periods of hypomanic mood for at least 2 years.

Risk Factors/Epidemiology. Many of the patients have interpersonal and marital difficulties. It frequently coexists with borderline personality disorder and is seen more frequently in women. Many of the patients with this disorder have family histories of bipolar disorder. Alcohol and substance abuse are common.

Treatment. Antimanic drugs such as lithium, carbamazepine, and valproic acid are typically the drugs of choice. Psychotherapy will focus on helping the patients gain insight into their illness and how to cope with it.

Differential Diagnosis

- *Medical:* Seizures, substances, and medications
- *Mental:* Other mood disorders, personality disorders. medications again

MAJOR DEPRESSIVE DISORDER WITH SEASONAL PATTERN

A young woman from Minnesota complains of depressed mood and sleep disturbances every winter. Her symptoms resolve in the spring and summer.

Definition. A disorder characterized by depressive symptoms found during winter months and absent during summer months. Believed to be caused by abnormal melatonin metabolism (decreased MSH).

Treatment. Phototherapy

GRIEF, POSTPARTUM DEPRESSION, DEATH AND DYING

Grief

Table I-5-1. Grief Versus Depression

Grief or Bereavement	Depression
Sadness, tearfulness, decreased sleep, decreased appetite, decreased interest in the world	Sadness, tearfulness, decreased sleep, decreased appetite, decreased interest in the world
Symptoms wax and wane	Symptoms pervasive and unremitting
Shame and guilt less common	Shame and guilt are common
Threaten suicide less often	Threaten suicide more often
Symptoms can last up to one year	Symptoms continue for more than one year
Usually return to baseline level of functioning within 2 months	Patients do not return to baseline level of functioning
Treatment includes supportive psychotherapy	Treatment includes antidepressant medication

Peripartum Mood Disorders

Table I-5-2. Postpartum Reactions

Onset	Disorder	Symptoms	Mother's Feelings Toward Baby	Treatment
Onset of mood symptoms within 2 wks after delivery	Postpartum blues or baby blues	Sadness, mood lability, tearfulness	No negative feelings	Supportive, usually self-limited
Onset of mood symptoms occurs during pregnancy or in the 4 wks following delivery	Depressive disorder with peripartum onset	Depressed mood, weight changes, sleep disturbances, and excessive anxiety	May have negative feelings toward baby	Antidepressant medications
Onset of mood and/or psychotic symptoms occurs during pregnancy or in the 4 wks following delivery	Bipolar disorder with peripartum onset Brief psychotic disorder with peripartum onset	Symptoms of depression, mania along with delusions, hallucinations and thoughts of harm	May have thoughts of harming baby	Antipsychotic medication, lithium, and possible antidepressant

Death and Dying

Based on the stages identified by Elisabeth Kubler-Ross. She believed dying patients did not follow a regular series of responses that could be easily identified. She believed most individuals experience stages that are common reactions to death. These stages do not have to occur in order.

Stage 1: Shock and denial

Stage 2: Anger

Stage 3: Bargaining

Stage 4: Depression

Stage 5: Acceptance

Review Questions

1. A 50-year-old woman is taken to the hospital after neighbors find her wandering the streets mumbling to herself and gesturing. When approached, she begins to cry and expresses thoughts about hurting herself. Examination reveals scratch marks on both her forearms and questionable lacerations on her throat. When questioned, she reports feeling depressed since her husband died 5 months ago. She reports a decrease in concentration and feelings of helplessness, hopelessness, and anhedonia, which resulted in her quitting her job and staying at home. She now has begun to hear her husband's voice asking her to "join" him. Which of the following would be the next step in management?

   (A) Begin a trial of antidepressant medications

   (B) Refer to psychiatry

   (C) Refer for electroconvulsive therapy

   (D) Assess for thoughts about suicide

   (E) Refer to the outpatient department for follow-up

2. Assuming you decide to begin treatment, which of the following is most indicated as initial treatment?

   (A) Individual psychotherapy

   (B) Behavioral therapy

   (C) Fluoxetine

   (D) Risperidone

   (E) Phenelzine

3. A 32-year-old woman was recently diagnosed with advanced breast cancer. Which of the following reactions would you expect to see first?

   (A) Shock and denial

   (B) Anger

   (C) Bargaining

   (D) Depression

   (E) Any of the above

1. **Answer: D.** The most important thing to assess in patients suffering from depression is their suicidal status, which of course determines her prognosis and whether or not you will admit her to the hospital for treatment. You will probably begin a course of pharm-acotherapy, but you need to assess suicidal status first. "Refer to psychiatry" will always be wrong on a test, given that you need to know what to do in these situations. Electroconvulsive therapy might be indicated in her condition but is usually not the first line of treatment.

2. **Answer: D.** Patients with both mood and psychotic symptoms respond to both antidepressants as well as to antipsychotic medication. However, you must treat the worst symptom first. In this case, the antipsychotic would be most indicated to reduce her psychotic symptoms. Choice D is an atypical antipsychotic medication with minimal side effects.

3. **Answer: E.** Because the stages can occur in any order, any one of the above is the answer.

Schizophrenia and Other Psychotic Disorders

5

Definition. Schizophrenia is a thought disorder that impairs judgment, behavior, and ability to interpret reality. Symptoms must be present for at least 6 months to be able to make a diagnosis.

Risk Factors/Etiology. Men have an earlier onset, usually at age 15–25. Many theories have evolved regarding the cause of schizophrenia.

- Schizophrenia has been associated with high levels of dopamine and abnormalities in serotonin.
- Because there is an increase in the number of schizophrenics born in the winter and early spring, many believe it may be viral in origin.

Schizophrenia is more prevalent in the low socioeconomic status (SES) groups, either as a result of downward drift or social causation.

Prevalence

General population........... 1% One schizophrenic parent................12%

Monozygotic twin........... 47% Two schizophrenic parents 40%

Dizygotic twin................ 12% First-degree relative.........................12%

Second-degree relative 5–6%

Physical and Psychiatric Presenting Symptoms

- Hallucinations (mostly auditory)
- Delusions (mostly bizarre)
- Disorganized speech or behavior
- Catatonic behavior
- Negative symptoms
- Usually experience social and or occupational dysfunction
- Physical exam usually unremarkable, but may find saccadic eye movements, hypervigilance, etc.

Brain Imaging Findings

- *Computed tomography (CT):* Lateral and third **ventricular enlargement, reduction in cortical volume** (associated with the presence of negative symptoms, neuropsychiatric impairment, increased neurologic signs, and poor premorbid adjustment)
- *Magnetic Resonance Imaging (MRI):* Increased cerebral ventricles
- *Positron emission tomography (PET):* Hypoactivity of the frontal lobes and hyperactivity of the basal ganglia relative to the cerebral cortex

Psychologic Tests

- *IQ tests:* Will score lower on all IQ tests, maybe due to low intelligence at the onset or to deterioration as a result of the disease
- *Neuropsychologic:* Tests usually are consistent with bilateral frontal and temporal lobe dysfunction, including deficits in attention, retention time, and problem-solving ability.
- *Personality:* May give abnormal findings, such as bizarre ideations, etc.

Treatment. Hospitalization is usually recommended for either stabilization or safety of the patient. If you decide to use medications, antipsychotic medications are most indicated to help control both positive and negative symptoms. If no response, consider using clozapine after other medications have failed. The suggested psychotherapy will be supportive psychotherapy with the primary aim of having the patient understand that the therapist is trustworthy and has an understanding of the patient, no matter how bizarre.

Differential Diagnosis

- *Substance-induced:* Psychostimulants, hallucinogens, alcohol hallucinosis, barbiturate withdrawal, etc. Consider urine drug screen to rule out.
- *Epilepsy:* Temporal lobe epilepsy
- *Other psychotic disorders:* Schizoaffective, schizophreniform, brief reactive psychosis, delusional disorder
- *Malingering and factitious disorder:* Must assess whether the patient is in control of the symptoms and whether there is an obvious gain
- *Mood disorders:* Look at duration of mood symptoms; these tend to be brief in schizophrenia.
- *Medical:* HIV, steroids, tumors, CVAs, etc. Need medical work-up to rule out.
- *Personality disorders:* Schizotypal, schizoid, and borderline personality disorders have the most similar symptoms. Must look at duration of symptoms as well as patient's level of functioning.

OTHER PSYCHOTIC DISORDERS

Brief Psychotic Disorder

A 35-year-old female Chinese immigrant is brought in by neighbors after she was found wandering in the streets yelling out someone's name. She appears disheveled and grossly disorganized. You learn that she arrived in the U.S. several days ago and upon her arrival, witnessed the death of her 3-year-old son. While in the waiting room, she appears to be responding to internal stimuli.

Presenting Symptoms

- Hallucinations
- Delusions
- Disorganized speech
- Grossly disorganized or catatonic behavior
- Symptoms more than one day but less than 30 days

Risk Factors. Seen most frequently in the low socioeconomic status as well as in those who have preexisting personality disorders or the presence of psychological stressors.

Treatment. Hospitalization is warranted if the patient is acutely psychotic, to assure the safety of her/himself or of others. Pharmacotherapy will include both antipsychotics and benzodiazepines. The benzodiazepines may be used for short-term treatment of psychotic symptoms.

Schizophreniform Disorder

Mrs. Jones is evaluated at a nearby clinic after she was noticed to be acting inappropriately at work. According to her coworkers, she began acting strangely 3 months ago. At that time she began wearing a hard hat to work and when asked why, replied, "I will not let you read my mind." She also believed that others were talking about her and routinely asked them to stop. On several occasions, she had to be escorted out of the room because she started to argue with others whom she believed were controlling her mind.

Presenting Symptoms

- Hallucinations
- Delusions
- Disorganized speech
- Grossly disorganized or catatonic behavior
- Negative symptoms
- Social and/or occupational dysfunction
- Symptoms are present more than one month but less than 6 months
- Most of the patients return to their baseline level of functioning

Risk Factors. Suicide is a risk factor given that the patient is likely to have a depressive episode after the psychotic symptoms resolve.

Treatment. Must assess whether the patient needs hospitalization, to assure safety of patient and/or others.

Antipsychotic medication is indicated for a 3–6-month course. Individual psychotherapy may be indicated to help the patient assimilate the psychotic experience into his/her life.

Schizoaffective Disorder

A 25-year-old woman is found walking nude in the shopping mall. When asked why, she replies, "I am making it easy for others to have sex with me since I know they all want me." She states she heard a voice telling her she was irresistible and everyone wanted her. When she speaks, she cannot focus on one topic at a time. Her mood is euphoric and her affect labile. She recounts an episode last year, where, although she did not have an elevated or depressed mood, she heard voices she could not describe and believed others were following her. These symptoms lasted for 6+ months and caused her to lose her job.

Presenting Symptoms

- Uninterrupted period of symptoms meeting criteria for major depressive episode, manic episode, or mixed episode
- Symptoms for schizophrenia
- Delusions or hallucinations for at least 2 weeks in the absence of mood symptoms

Prognosis. Better prognosis than patients with schizophrenia. Worse prognosis than patients with affective disorders.

Treatment. First determine if hospitalization is necessary. Use antidepressant medications and/ or anticonvulsants to control the mood symptoms. If not effective, consider antipsychotics to help control the ongoing symptoms.

Delusional Disorder

Mr. Smith has been married for 10 years, and during most of those years he believed his wife was trying to poison him to get his money. He frequently complains of stomach pain, which he believes is due to the poison in the food. His thoughts are logical and coherent. He denies any hallucinations. His wife, an independently wealthy woman, does not understand her husband's logic because she has more money than he does.

Presenting Symptoms

- Nonbizarre delusions for at least 1 month
- No impairment in level of functioning
- The patients are usually reliable unless it is in relationship to their delusions.
- Types include erotomanic, jealous, grandiose, somatic, mixed, unspecified.

Risk Factors. Mean age of onset is about age 40. Seen more commonly in women, and most are married and employed. Has been associated with low socioeconomic status as well as recent immigration. Can usually see conditions in limbic system or basal ganglia, if medical causes are determined to be the cause of the delusions.

Treatment. Outpatient treatment is usually preferred, but the patient may need hospitalization while you rule out medical causes. Pharmacotherapy consists of antipsychotic medications, but studies indicate that many patients do not respond to treatment. Individual psychotherapy is recommended, having the patient trust the physician to point out how the delusions interfere with normal life.

Review Questions

1. A 23-year-old woman was seen today after she complained that her neighbors were talking about her. According to the neighbors, her behavior started 3 weeks ago after she was involved in a car accident. She was not injured in the accident. Since then, she has been following the neighbors for several days and harassing them at work. She believes that the neighbors are putting poison in her food and want to kill her. When asked why, she is unable to give a clear explanation but insists that what she is saying is true. She states that the voice in her head told her it is true and that you should stop asking questions. While in the waiting room, you observe her to be dressed bizarrely and laughing inappropriately. Which of the following is most indicated in management?

   (A) Haloperidol

   (B) Clozapine

   (C) Lorazepam

   (D) Risperidone

   (E) Fluphenazine decanoate

2. If her symptoms do not improve within the next week, which of the following is she at greatest risk of developing?

   (A) Schizophrenia, paranoid type

   (B) Schizoaffective disorder

   (C) Schizophreniform disorder

   (D) Schizotypal personality disorder

   (E) Delusional disorder

---

1. **Answer: D.** The patient clearly has psychotic symptoms; therefore, you would want to give her medication with the fewest side effects. Choices A and E are typical antipsychotics with many side effects. Choices B and D are atypical antipsychotics; however, clozapine is not used first line in the treatment of psychotic symptoms. Lorazepam is not an antipsychotic medication. However, it can be used in psychotic patients to reduce agitation.

2. **Answer: C.** Because her symptoms have occurred for only 3 weeks, this patient has a diagnosis of brief psychotic disorder. But should the symptoms persist for >1 month, her diagnosis would be schizophreniform disorder. Schizophrenia is given when the symptoms are present for >6 months.

Anxiety Disorders 6

Definition. Anxiety is a syndrome with psychologic and physiologic components. Psychologic components include worry that is difficult to control, hypervigilance and restlessness, difficulty concentrating, and sleep disturbance. Physiologic components include autonomic hyperactivity and motor tension.

Risk Factors/Etiology. Psychodynamic theory posits that anxiety occurs when instinctual drives are thwarted. Behavioral theory states that anxiety is a conditioned response to environmental stimuli originally paired with a feared situation. Biologic theories implicate various neurotransmitters (especially gamma-aminobutyric acid [GABA], norepinephrine, and serotonin) and various CNS structures (especially reticular activating system and limbic system).

PANIC DISORDER

Definition. Recurrent, unexpected panic attacks are present. Panic attacks are attacks of intense anxiety that often include marked physical symptoms, such as tachycardia, hyperventilation, dizziness, and sweating. Attacks followed by 1 month of fear of having no attacks, changing behavior, etc.

Risk Factors/Etiology. History associated with panic disorder includes separations during childhood and interpersonal loss in adulthood. A majority of individuals with panic disorder, unlike other individuals, have panic symptoms in response to "panicogens" (lactate CO_2, yohimbine, caffeine, and other substances). Studies of twins suggest a genetic component.

Presenting Symptoms

- *Prevalence:* 2% of the population. Occurs at a 1:2 male-to-female ratio.
- *Onset:* Often during the third decade
- *Course:* Severity of symptoms may wax and wane, and may be associated with intercurrent stressors.
- *Key symptoms:* Attacks usually last a few minutes.
- *Associated problems:* Depression, generalized anxiety, and substance abuse
- *Agoraphobia:* Fear or avoidance of places from which escape would be difficult in the event of panic symptoms (public places, being outside alone, public transportation, crowds). More common in women. Often leads to severe restrictions on the individual's travel and daily routine.

Treatment. Pharmacologic interventions include SSRIs, alprazolam, clonazepam, imipramine, and MAOIs (e.g., phenelzine). Psychotherapeutic interventions include relaxation training for panic attacks and systematic desensitization for agoraphobic symptoms.

PHOBIC DISORDERS

Definition. Irrational fear and avoidance of objects and situations

Types of Phobias

- **Specific phobia:** Fear or avoidance of objects or situations other than agoraphobia or social phobia. Commonly involves animals (e.g., carnivores, spiders), natural environments (e.g., storms), injury (e.g., injections, blood), and situations (e.g., heights, darkness).

- **Social anxiety disorder:** Fear of humiliation or embarrassment in either general or specific social situations (e.g., public speaking, "stage fright," urinating in public restrooms).

Treatment. Cognitive-behavioral therapies for phobias include systematic desensitization and assertiveness training. Pharmacotherapy includes SSRIs, buspirone, and beta-blockers (for stage fright).

OBSESSIVE-COMPULSIVE DISORDER (OCD)

Definition. OCD is characterized by recurrent obsessions or compulsions that are recognized by the individual as unreasonable. Obsessions are anxiety-provoking, intrusive thoughts, commonly concerning contamination, doubt, guilt, aggression, and sex. Compulsions are peculiar behaviors that reduce anxiety, commonly hand-washing, organizing, checking, counting, and praying.

Risk Factors/Etiology. May be associated with abnormalities of serotonin metabolism

Presenting Symptoms

- *Prevalence:* 2% of population. Occurs at a 1:1 male-to-female ratio.
- Some evidence of heritability
- *Onset:* Insidious and occurs during childhood, adolescence, or early adulthood
- *Course:* Symptoms usually wax and wane, and depression, other anxieties, and substance abuse are common.

Physical Examination. Chapped hands when hand-washing compulsion is present.

Treatment. Behavioral psychotherapies are relaxation training, guided imagery, exposure, paradoxical intent, response prevention, thought-stopping techniques, and modeling. Pharmacotherapy includes selective serotonin reuptake inhibitors, TCAs, MAOIs, and SNRIs.

ACUTE STRESS DISORDER/POST-TRAUMATIC STRESS DISORDER

Definition. These disorders are characterized by severe anxiety symptoms and follow a threatening event that caused feelings of fear, helplessness, or horror.

- When this anxiety lasts <1 month (but >2 days) and symptoms occur within 1 month of stressor, it is diagnosed as **acute stress disorder (ASD)**.

- When the anxiety lasts >1 month, it is diagnosed as **post traumatic stress disorder (PTSD)**.

Risk Factors/Etiology. Traumatic events precipitate ASD and PTSD. Premorbid factors, such as personality traits, play an uncertain role.

Presenting Symptoms

- May occur at any age. About 50% of cases resolve within 3 months.
- Usually begin immediately after trauma, but may occur after months or years.
- Three key symptom groups
    - Reexperiencing of traumatic event: dreams, flashbacks, or intrusive recollections
    - Avoidance of stimuli associated with the trauma or numbing of general responsiveness
    - Increased arousal: anxiety, sleep disturbances, hypervigilance
- Anxiety, depression, impulsivity, and emotional lability are common.
- *"Survivor guilt":* A feeling of irrational guilt about an event sometimes occurs.

Treatment. Counseling after a stressful event may prevent PTSD from developing. Group psychotherapy with other survivors is helpful. Pharmacotherapy includes SSRIs, other antidepressants, and benzodiazepines. Prazosin has been used to reduce nightmares.

GENERALIZED ANXIETY DISORDER

Definition. Excessive, poorly controlled anxiety about life circumstances that continues for more than 6 months. Both psychologic and physiologic symptoms of anxiety are present. General worry is accompanied by somatic symptoms such as irritability, decreased sleep, and poor concentration.

Risk Factors/Etiology. May be a genetic predisposition for an anxiety trait

Presenting Symptoms

- *Prevalence:* 5% of the population. Occurs at a 2:3 male-to-female ratio.
- *Onset:* Often during childhood but can occur later
- *Course:* Usually chronic, but symptoms worsen with stress
- *Associated problems:* Depression, somatic symptoms, and substance abuse

Treatment. Behavioral psychotherapy includes relaxation training and biofeedback. Pharmacotherapy includes SSRIs, venlafaxine, buspirone, and benzodiazepines.

Review Question

A 31-year-old local politician has a sudden onset of extreme anxiety, tremulousness, and diaphoresis immediately before his first scheduled appearance on national television, and he is unable to go on the air. For the next week he is paralyzed by fear each time he faces an audience, and he cancels all of his scheduled public appearances.

Which of the following is the most likely diagnosis?

(A) Acute stress disorder

(B) Adjustment disorder with anxious mood

(C) Panic disorder

(D) Social anxiety disorder

(E) Specific phobia

Answer: D. This presentation is most suggestive of social anxiety disorder. In this case, exposure to public speaking precipitated intense anxiety. Panic disorder is also characterized by intense anxiety attacks; however, there is no clear precipitant. Specific phobia, situational type, is a less likely diagnosis, because there is no specific cause of the fear other than social exposure. Acute stress disorder is characterized by the presence of intrusive recollections and emotional numbing that follow a life-threatening event. Adjustment disorder with anxious mood is characterized by an adaptation problem that follows a psychologic stressor, of which there is no evidence in this case.

Used with permission from Williams & Wilkins, *Board Review Series: Psychiatry*, 1997.

Somatic Symptom and Related Disorders

7

Definition. Somatoform disorders are characterized by the presentation of physical symptoms with no medical explanation(s). The symptoms are severe enough to interfere with the patient's ability to function in social or occupational activities.

SOMATIC SYMPTOM DISORDER

> Mrs. Smith has been married for approximately 10 years, and during all of those years she remembers being sick all of the time. According to her husband, she constantly takes medications for all of her ailments. She has visited numerous physicians and none have been able to correctly diagnose her condition. Today she presents in your office complaining of shortness of breath, chest pain, abdominal pain, back pain, double vision, difficulty walking due to weakness in her legs, headaches, constipation, bloating, decreased libido, and tingling in her fingers.

Definition. A disorder where one or more somatic symptoms that are distressing result in problems in functioning.

Risk Factors/Etiology. Somatization disorder affects women more than men and is usually inversely related to SES. Usually begins by the age of 30. Data suggest that there may be a genetic linkage to the disorder. Within families, male relatives tend to have antisocial personality disorder, whereas female relatives tend to have histrionic personality disorder.

Physical and Psychiatric Presenting Symptoms
- Many physical symptoms affecting many organ systems
- Excessive thoughts, feelings, or behaviors related to the somatic symptoms
- Long, complicated medical histories
- Interpersonal and psychologic problems are usually present.
- Patients will usually seek out treatment and have significant impairment in their level of functioning.
- Commonly associated with major depressive disorder, personality disorders, substance-related disorders, generalized anxiety disorders, and phobias

Treatment. Must have a single identified physician as the primary caretaker. Patient should be seen during regularly scheduled brief monthly visits. Should increase the patient's awareness of the possibility that the symptoms are psychological in nature. Individual psychotherapy is needed to help patients cope with their symptoms and develop other ways of expressing their feelings.

Differential Diagnosis

- *Medical:* MS, myasthenia gravis, SLE, AIDS, thyroid disorders, and chronic systemic infections
- *Psychiatric:* Major depression, generalized anxiety disorder, schizophrenia

CONVERSION DISORDER

A recently married woman presents to the emergency department unable to move her lower extremities. A full workup is done, and no abnormalities are found. When further questioned, she reports being beaten by her husband that morning.

Definition. A disorder in which the individual experiences one or more neurologic symptoms that cannot be explained by any medical or neurologic disorder.

Risk Factors/Etiology. Seen more frequently in young women. Also more common among the lower SES, rural populations, low IQs, and military personnel. Commonly associated with passive-aggressive, dependent, antisocial, and histrionic personality disorder.

Psychiatric and Physical Presenting Symptoms

- One or two neurologic symptoms affecting voluntary or sensory function
- Must have psychologic factors associated with the onset or exacerbation of the symptoms
- Mutism, blindness, and paralysis are the most common symptoms.
- *Sensory system:* Anesthesia and paresthesia
- *Motor system:* Abnormal movements, gait disturbance, weakness, paralysis, tics, jerks, etc.
- *Seizure system:* Pseudoseizures
- *Primary gain:* Keeps internal conflicts outside patient's awareness
- *Secondary gain:* Benefits received from being "sick"
- *La belle indifference:* Patient seems unconcerned about impairment.
- *Identification:* Patients usually model their behavior on someone who is important to them.

Treatment. Psychotherapy to establish a caring relationship with treater and focus on stress and coping skills. Brief monthly visits with partial physical examinations.

Differential Diagnosis

- *Neurologic:* Dementia, tumors, basal ganglia disease, and optic neuritis
- *Psychiatric:* Schizophrenia, depressive disorders, anxiety disorders, factitious
- *Other:* Malingering

ILLNESS ANXIETY DISORDER

A 22-year-old woman presents to the doctor convinced that she has a brain tumor. She reports frequent headaches that are not alleviated with aspirin. She has been to numerous physicians and all have told her that there is nothing wrong with her. She expects that you can help her because she knows that there is something wrong and that you can adequately treat her condition.

Definition. A disorder characterized by the patient's belief that he/she has some specific disease. Despite constant reassurance, the patient's belief remains the same. Symptoms must occur for >6 months.

Risk Factors/Etiology. Men and women are affected equally. Most common onset is between the ages of 20 and 30.

Physical and Psychiatric Presenting Symptoms

- Preoccupation with diseases
- The preoccupation persists despite constant reassurance by physicians.
- The belief is not delusional.
- The preoccupation affects the individual's level of functioning.
- Duration at least 6 months

Treatment. Psychotherapy to help relieve stress and help cope with illness. Frequent, regularly scheduled visits to patient's medical doctor(s).

BODY DYSMORPHIC DISORDER

The mother of a 20-year-old man presents to your office in tears. She insists that you come to her house and see her son, who has been homebound for several years. She explains that her son refuses to leave the house because he believes he is ugly and people will laugh at him. He feels deformed and refuses to let others see him. When you arrive at the house, you find an attractive young man with no observable deformities.

Definition. A disorder characterized by the belief that some body part is abnormal, defective, or misshapen.

Risk Factors/Etiology. Affects women more than men, typically ages 15–20. These women are unlikely to be married. Other disorders that may be found include depressive disorders, anxiety disorders, and psychotic disorders. Family history of depressive disorders and OCDs. May involve serotonergic systems.

Physical and Psychiatric Presenting Symptoms

- Most common concerns involve facial flaws
- Constant mirror-checking
- Attempt to hide the alleged deformity

- Housebound
- Avoids social situations
- Causes impairment in their level of functioning

Treatment. Individual psychotherapy to help deal with stress of alleged imperfections as well as reality testing. Pharmacotherapy may include the use of SSRIs, TCAs, or MAOIs.

Differential Diagnosis

- *Medical:* Some types of brain damage, such as neglect syndrome
- *Psychiatric:* Anorexia, narcissistic personality disorder, OCD, schizophrenia, delusional disorder

FACTITIOUS DISORDER

A 2-year-old girl was hospitalized after her mother complained that the girl had multiple episodes of apnea in the middle of the night. The mother was given an apnea monitor to take home and when she returned, there were numerous episodes registering on the monitor. While in the hospital, the girl had no episodes of apnea. However, shortly after her mother's visit, there were numerous episodes recorded on the monitor.

Definition. A disorder characterized by the conscious production of signs and symptoms of both medical and mental disorders. The main objective is to assume the sick role and eventually hospitalization. Usually diagnosed with physical or psychological symptoms or both. Consists of 2 main types: **imposed on self** and **imposed on others**.

Etiology. Seen more commonly in women and in hospital and health care workers. As children, many of the patients suffered abuse that resulted in frequent hospitalizations, thus their need to assume the sick role.

Physical and Psychiatric Presenting Symptoms

- Typically demand treatment when in the hospital
- If tests return negative, they tend to accuse doctors and threaten litigation.
- Become angry when confronted

Treatment. Usually involves management rather than cure. Must be aware of countertransference when the physician suspects factitious disorder.

Differential Diagnosis. Psychiatric: Other somatoform disorders, antisocial personality disorder, histrionic personality disorder, schizophrenia, substance abuse, malingering, and Ganser's syndrome

MALINGERING

A 40-year-old homeless man presents to the hospital on a cold night complaining of auditory hallucinations telling him to kill himself. When asked about past psychiatric history, he is unable to give any detailed information. He seems concerned about being admitted immediately and refuses all medications, when offered.

Definition. Characterized by the conscious production of signs and symptoms for an obvious gain (money, avoidance of work, free bed and board, etc.). It is not a mental disorder.

Risk Factors/Etiology. Seen more frequently in men, especially in prisons, factories, the military, etc.

Physical and Psychiatric Presenting Symptoms

- Most express subjective symptoms.
- Tend to complain a lot and exaggerate its effect on their functioning and lives
- Preoccupied more with rewards than with alleviation of symptoms

Treatment. Allow the patient to save face by not confronting the patient and by allowing the physician–patient relationship to work. If confronted, patient will become angry and more guarded and suspicious.

Differential Diagnosis. Psychiatric: somatoform disorders

Review Question

A 40-year-old woman presents to your office and demands to be seen immediately. She schedules appointments to see you on a regular basis as well as irregularly. She routinely goes to the emergency department when she knows you are in the hospital. She calls your service every night and demands that you call her at home. Her frequent complaints include headache, shortness of breath, double vision, burning at urination, weakness in her arms and legs, tingling in her fingers, and palpitations. All of her medical workups have been negative so far.

Which of the following would be the next step in management?

(A) Tell her it is all in her head

(B) Assure her there is nothing wrong with her

(C) Refer her to a psychiatrist

(D) Begin a trial of lorazepam

(E) Schedule regular office visits

Answer: E. Patients with somatic symptom disorder should have only one physician, and that physician must see the patient on a regular basis given that there might be something physically wrong in the future. Also, by limiting the patient's care to one physician, the likelihood of unnecessary tests and treatment is reduced.

Neurocognitive Disorders 8

Cognition includes memory, language, orientation, judgment, problem solving, interpersonal relationships, and performance of actions. Cognitive disorders have problems in these areas as well as behavioral symptoms.

Definition. Characterized by the syndromes of delirium, neurocognitive disorder, and amnesia, which are caused by general medical conditions, substances, or both.

Risk Factors/Etiology. Very young or advanced age, debilitation, presence of specific general medical conditions, sustained or excessive exposure to a variety of substances.

Presenting Symptoms (Key Symptoms)

- Memory impairment, especially recent memory
- **Aphasia:** Failure of language function
- **Apraxia:** Failure of ability to execute complex motor behaviors
- **Agnosia:** Failure to recognize or identify people or objects
- **Disturbances in executive function:** Impairment in the ability to think abstractly and plan such activities as organizing, shopping, and maintaining a home

DELIRIUM

Definition. Delirium is characterized by prominent disturbances in alertness, as well as confusion and a short, fluctuating course. It is caused by acute metabolic problems or substance intoxication.

Risk Factors/Etiology. Commonly associated with general medical conditions such as systemic infections, metabolic disorders, hepatic/renal diseases, seizures, head trauma. Also associated with high, sustained, or rapidly decreasing levels of many drugs, especially in the elderly and severely ill.

Presenting Symptoms. Delirium occurs in >40% of elderly, hospitalized patients. Key symptoms include agitation or stupor, fear, emotional lability, hallucinations, delusions, and disturbed psychomotor activity.

Physical Examination. Motor abnormalities commonly present, include incoordination, tremor, asterixis, and nystagmus. Incontinence is common. There is often evidence of underlying general medical conditions or substance-specific syndromes.

Diagnostic Tests. EEG often shows generalized slowing of activity, fast-wave activity, or focal abnormalities. Abnormal findings from neuroimaging and neuropsychiatric testing may be present.

Treatment. Correction of physiologic problems is essential. Frequent orientation and reassurance are helpful. Consider protective use of physical restraints and antipsychotic medications.

Differential Diagnosis. Neurocognitive disorder, substance intoxication or withdrawal, and psychotic disorders are the major rule-outs.

NEUROCOGNITIVE DISORDER

Definition. Neurocognitive disorder is characterized by slight (mild) or prominent (severe) memory disturbances coupled with other cognitive disturbances that are present even in the absence of delirium. It is caused by CNS damage and likely to have a protracted course.

Risk Factors/Etiology.

- Neurodegenerative disease such as Alzheimer, Parkinson, Huntington, Pick, and other fronto-temporal degeneration, and Creutzfeldt-Jakob disease are common causes.

- Cerebrovascular disease, intracranial processes such as CNS infections (e.g., HIV), traumatic brain injuries, radiation, and/or tumors should be considered.

- Seizure disorders, metabolic disorders (e.g., disease of protein, lipid, and carbohydrate metabolism; diseases of myelin; Wilson disease; uremic encephalopathy), and endocrinopathies (e.g., hypothyroidism) are often associated with neurocognitive disorder.

- Nutritional deficiencies, including beriberi (thiamine [vitamin B1] deficiency), pellagra (niacin deficiency), and/or pernicious anemia (cobalamin [vitamin B12] deficiency), should be considered.

- Toxins that cause neurocognitive disorder include alcohol, inhalants, sedative–hypnotics, anxiolytics, anticonvulsants, antineoplastic medications, heavy metals, insecticides, and solvents.

Prevalence. 5% of the population age >65 and >20% of the population age >85

Heritability. Some types of neurodegenerative neurocognitive disorders (e.g., Huntington disease).

Key Symptoms. Increasing disorientation, anxiety, depression, emotional lability, personality disturbances, hallucinations, and delusions

Associated Findings. Abnormal findings from neuroimaging and neuropsychiatric testing.

Course. Depending on the etiology, function may stabilize or deteriorate further.

Physical Examination. Evidence of CNS motor pathology is often present. There may be evidence of underlying general medical conditions or substance-specific syndromes.

Diagnostic Tests. EEG may show specific focal abnormalities. Neuroimaging and neuropsychiatric testing may show specific abnormal findings. Folstein Mini-Mental Status Exam is used to detect neurocognitive disorder. Basic laboratory examination for neurocognitive disorder includes B12 and folate levels, RPR, CBC with SMA, and thyroid function tests.

Treatment. Correction or amelioration of underlying pathology is essential. Medication that further impairs cognition should be avoided. Provision of familiar surroundings, reassurance, and emotional support is often helpful.

Differential Diagnosis. Delirium and less severe, age-related cognitive decline must be ruled out.

Specific Neurocognitive Disorders

All neurocognitive disorders may be mild or severe.

Neurocognitive disorder due to Alzheimer disease

- Occupy more than 50% of nursing-home beds
- Found in 50–60% of patients with neurocognitive disorder
- Risk factors: Female, family history, head trauma, Down syndrome
- Neuroanatomic findings: Cortical atrophy, flattened sulci, and enlarged ventricles
- Histopathology: Senile plaques (amyloid deposits), neurofibrillary tangles, neuronal loss, synaptic loss, and granulovacuolar degeneration of neurons
- Associated with chromosome #21 (gene for the amyloid precursor protein)
- Decreased Ach and NE
- Deterioration is generally gradual; average duration from onset to death is ~8 years.
- Focal neurologic symptoms are rare.
- Treatment includes long-acting cholinesterase inhibitors such as donepezil, rivastigmine, galantamine, and memantine..
- Antipsychotic medications may be helpful when psychotic symptoms present but contraindicated to control behavior.

Vascular neurocognitive disorder (multi-infarct neurocognitive disorder)

- Found in 15–30% of patients with neurocognitive disorder
- Risk factors: Male, advanced age, hypertension, or other cardiovascular disorders
- Affects small and medium-sized vessels
- Examination may reveal carotid bruits, fundoscopic abnormalities, and enlarged cardiac chambers.
- MRI may reveal hyperintensities and focal atrophy suggestive of old infarctions.
- Deterioration may be stepwise or gradual, depending on underlying pathology.
- Focal neurologic symptoms (pseudobulbar palsy, dysarthria, and dysphagia are most common)
- Abnormal reflexes and gait disturbance are often present.
- Treatment is directed toward the underlying condition and lessening cell damage.
- Control of risk factors such as hypertension, smoking, diabetes, hypercholesterolemia, and hyperlipidemia is useful.

Table I-8-1. Alzheimer Versus Vascular Neurocognitive Disorder

Alzheimer	Vascular
Women	Men
Older age of onset	Younger than Alzheimer patients
Chromosome 21	Hypertension
Linear or progressive deterioration	Stepwise or patchy deterioration
No focal deficits	Focal deficits
Supportive treatment	Treat underlying condition

Frontotemporal neurocognitive disorder (Pick disease)

- Neuroanatomic findings: Atrophy in the frontal and temporal lobes
- Histopathology: Pick bodies (intraneuronal argentophilic inclusions) and Pick cells (swollen neurons) in affected areas of the brain
- Etiology is unknown.
- Most common in men with family history of Pick disease
- Difficult to distinguish from Alzheimer's
- May see features of Klüver-Bucy syndrome (hypersexuality, hyperphagia, passivity)

Neurocognitive disorder due to Prion disease

- Rare spongiform encephalopathy is caused by a slow virus (prion).
- Presents with neurocognitive disorder, myoclonus, and EEG abnormalities (e.g., sharp, triphasic, synchronous discharges and, later, periodic discharges)
- Symptoms progress over months from vague malaise and personality changes to neurocognitive disorder and death.
- Findings include visual and gait disturbances, choreoathetosis or other abnormal movements, and myoclonus.
- Other prions that cause neurocognitive disorder (e.g., Kuru) may exist.

Neurocognitive disorder due to Huntington disease

- A rare, progressive neurodegenerative disease that involves loss of GABA-ergic neurons of the basal ganglia, manifested by choreoathetosis, neurocognitive disorder, and psychosis.
- Caused by a defect in an autosomal dominant gene located on chromosome 4
- Atrophy of the caudate nucleus, with resultant ventricular enlargement, is common.
- Clinical onset usually occurs at approximately age 40.
- Suicidal behavior is fairly common.

Neurocognitive disorder due to Parkinson disease

- Common, progressive, neurodegenerative disease involving loss of dopaminergic neurons in the substantia nigra
- Clinical onset is usually age 50–65.
- Motor symptoms include resting tremor, rigidity, bradykinesia, and gait disturbances.
- Neurocognitive disorder occurs in 40% of cases, and depressive symptoms are common.
- Destruction of dopaminergic neurons in the substantia nigra is a key pathogenic component and may be caused by multiple factors, including environmental toxins, infection, genetic predisposition, and aging.
- Treatment of Parkinson disease involves use of dopamine precursors (e.g., levodopa, carbidopa), dopamine agonists (e.g., bromocriptine), anticholinergic medications (e.g., benztropine, trihexyphenidyl), amantadine, and selegiline.
- Antiparkinsonian medications can produce personality changes, cognitive changes, and psychotic symptoms.

Neurocognitive disorder with Lewy bodies

Hallucinations, parkinsonian features, and extrapyramidal signs. Antipsychotic medications may worsen behavior. Patients typically have fluctuating cognition, as well as REM sleep behavior disorder.

Neurocognitive disorder due to HIV infection

- HIV directly and progressively destroys brain parenchyma.
- Becomes clinically apparent in at least 30% of individuals with AIDS, beginning with subtle personality changes.
- Diffuse and rapid multifocal destruction of brain structures occurs, and delirium is often present.
- Motor findings include gait disturbance, hypertonia and hyperreflexia, pathologic reflexes (e.g., frontal release signs), and oculomotor deficits.
- Mood disturbances in individuals with HIV infection are apathy, emotional liability, or behavioral disinhibition.

Wilson disease

- Ceruloplasmin deficiency
- Hepatolenticular degeneration
- Kayser-Fleischer rings in the eye
- Asterixis

Normal pressure hydrocephalus

- Enlarged ventricles
- Normal pressure
- Neurocognitive disorder, urinary incontinence, and gait apraxia
- Treatment includes shunt placement

Pseudodementia

- Typically seen in elderly patient who has a depressive disorder but appears to have symptoms of neurocognitive disorder; should improve after being treated with antidepressants
- Can usually date the onset of their symptoms

Table I-8-2. Pseudodementia versus Neurocognitive Disorder

Pseudodementia	Neurocognitive Disorder
Acute onset	Insidious onset
Family aware	Family unaware at first
Answers "I don't know" when asked questions	Confabulates when asked questions
Will talk about deficits when asked	Will minimize deficits
Treat with antidepressants	Will not improve with antidepressants

Note

(LBD) 1 yr $\leftarrow$ PD $\rightarrow$ 1 yr (PDD)

Table I-8-3. Delirium Versus Neurocognitive Disorder

Delirium	Neurocognitive Disorder
Acute onset	Insidious onset
Fluctuating course	Chronic course
Lasts days to weeks	Lasts months to years
Recent memory problems	Recent then remote memory problems
Disrupted sleep-wake cycle	Less disorientation at first
Disorientation	Normal sleep-wake cycle
Hallucinations common	Hallucinations, sundowning
Treat underlying condition	Supportive treatment

MILD NEUROCOGNITIVE DISORDER DUE TO SUBSTANCE/ MEDICATION OR ANOTHER MEDICAL CONDITION

Definition. Characterized by prominent memory impairment in the absence of disturbances in level of alertness or the other cognitive problems that are present with delirium or neurocognitive disorder.

Risk Factors/Etiology (General Medical Conditions). Commonly associated with bilateral damage to diencephalic and mediotemporal structures (e.g., mammillary bodies, fornix, hippocampus). It may also be caused by conditions such as thiamine deficiency associated with alcohol dependence, head trauma, cerebrovascular disease, hypoxia, local infection (e.g., herpes encephalitis), ablative surgical procedures, and seizures.

Risk Factors/Etiology (Substances). Alcohol is likely the most common cause.

Table I-8-4. Wernicke Versus Korsakoff Syndromes

	Wernicke	Korsakoff
Course	Acute	Chronic
Reversibility	Yes	No
Presentation	Ataxia, nystagmus, and ophthalmoplesia	Confusion, psychosis, anterograde and retrograde amnesia
Treatment	Thiamine	Thiamine

Physical Examination. Evidence of chronic alcohol abuse is often present.

Treatment. Correction of the underlying pathophysiology (e.g., administration of thiamine in alcohol-induced amnestic disorder) may be effective in reversing or slowing the progression of symptoms.

Differential Diagnosis. Delirium, neurocognitive disorder, and dissociative amnesia are the common rule-outs.

Review Question

A 65-year-old woman is found by the police in a filthy apartment after they were called by neighbors complaining of an unpleasant odor. Police find spoiled food in the kitchen, clogged sinks and toilets, and a severe infestation of cockroaches. The woman angrily refuses to leave with the police, stating that her neighbors have threatened her with attack and she fears that they will rob her apartment in her absence. Emergency room assessment reveals a very frail and unkempt woman who is completely alert and attentive. She believes it is 10 years earlier than it actually is, and she seems confused about her current finances and social contacts. She is unable to give the current addresses or phone numbers of her children and cannot find her phone book or purse. Physical exam is WNL.

Which of the following disturbances is the most likely diagnosis?

(A)   Vascular neurocognitive disorder

(B)   Wernicke's syndrome

(C)   Pseudodementia

(D)   Delirium

(E)   Neurocognitive disorder due to Alzheimer's disease

Answer: E. The woman presents with evidence of memory disturbance and severe problems managing her activities. This presentation is most consistent with neurocognitive disorder, which is characterized by memory impairment and other cognitive deficits. Delirium is characterized by problems with arousal and attention in addition to cognitive disturbances. Wernicke's is a less likely diagnosis because no cognitive disturbances other than memory impairment are present in this patient. Pseudodementia occurs quickly and patients are aware of the symptoms. Vascular neurocognitive disorder will often show motor deficits on physical exam.

Used with permission from Williams & Wilkins, *Board Review Series: Psychiatry*, 1997.

Dissociative Disorders 9

Dissociation is the fragmentation or separation of aspects of consciousness, including memory, identity, and perception. Some degree of dissociation is always present; however, if an individual's consciousness becomes too fragmented, it may pathologically interfere with the sense of self and ability to adapt. Presenting complaints and findings of dissociative disorders include amnesia, personality change, erratic behavior, odd inner experiences (e.g., flashbacks, déjà vu), and confusion.

DISSOCIATIVE AMNESIA AND DISSOCIATIVE AMNESIA WITH FUGUE

Definition. Significant episodes in which the individual is unable to recall important and often emotionally charged memories. Dissociative amnesia with fugue also involves purposeful travel or bewildered wandering.

Risk Factors/Etiology. Psychological stress. More common in women and younger adults. Onset is usually detected retrospectively by the discovery of memory gaps of extremely variable duration.

Symptoms. Amnesia that may be general or selective for certain events.

Course. The amnesia may suddenly or gradually remit, particularly when the traumatic circumstance resolves, or may become chronic.

Associated Problems. Mood disorders, conversion disorder, and personality disorders are commonly present.

Treatment. Diagnostic evaluation for general medical conditions (e.g., head trauma, seizures, cerebrovascular disease) or substances (e.g., anxiolytic and hypnotic medications, alcohol) that may cause amnesia. Hypnosis, suggestion, and relaxation techniques are helpful. The patient should be removed from stressful situations when possible. Psychotherapy should be directed at resolving underlying emotional stress.

Differential Diagnosis. Major rule-outs are amnestic disorder due to a general medical condition, substance-induced amnestic disorder, and other dissociative disorders.

DISSOCIATIVE IDENTITY DISORDER

Definition. Formerly called multiple personality disorder. Presence of multiple, distinct personalities that recurrently control the individual's behavior, accompanied by failure to recall important personal information.

Risk Factors/Etiology. Childhood sexual abuse has been postulated as a risk factor.

Prevalence. More common in women

Onset. Usually occult; clinical presentation is several years later when disturbances in interpersonal functioning are present.

Key Symptoms. Presence of distinct personalities is often subtle; in some cases, it is discovered only during treatment for associated symptoms.

Associated Problems. Chaotic interpersonal relationships, impulsivity and self-destructive behavior, suicide attempts, substance abuse

Comorbidity. Borderline personality disorder, PTSD, major depressive disorder and other mood disorders, substance-related disorders, sexual disorders, and eating disorders.

Course. Symptoms may fluctuate or be continuous.

Differential Diagnoses. Borderline personality disorder and other personality disorders, bipolar disorder with rapid cycling, factitious disorder, and malingering

Treatment. Psychotherapy to uncover psychologically traumatic memories and to resolve the associated emotional conflict

DEPERSONALIZATION AND DEREALIZATION DISORDER

Definition. Persistent or recurrent feeling of being detached from one's mental processes or body, accompanied by intact sense of reality

Risk Factors/Etiology. Psychologic stress

Prevalence. Episodes of depersonalization are common.

Onset. Usually in adolescence or early adulthood. Stressful events may precede the onset of the disorder.

Key Symptoms

- *Depersonalization:* Often described as an "out-of-body experience"
- *Derealization:* Perception of the environment is often distorted or strange during episodes of depersonalization, accompanied by a feeling of being detached from physical surroundings. *Jamais vu* (a sense of familiar things being strange), déjà vu (a sense of unfamiliar things being familiar), and other forms of perceptual distortion may occur.

Associated Symptoms. Are often during episodes

Treatment. Psychotherapy directed at decreasing anxiety

Differential Diagnosis. Major rule-outs are substance-induced mental disorders with dissociative symptoms, including intoxication, withdrawal, hallucinogen-induced persisting perceptual disorder, panic disorder, and PTSD.

Review Question

A 19-year-old man is brought to the emergency room by volunteers from a homeless shelter. The man claims that he cannot remember who he is. He says that he found himself in Los Angeles but that he cannot remember where he comes from, the circumstances of his trip, or any other information about his life. He has neither identification nor money, but he has a bus ticket from New York. Physical exam and laboratory testing are unremarkable.

Which of the following is the most likely diagnosis?

(A)   Depersonalization disorder

(B)   Dissociative amnesia

(C)   Dissociative amnesia fugue

(D)   Dissociative identity disorder

(E)   Substance-induced amnestic disorder

Answer: C. The symptoms of amnesia, unexplained travel, and identity confusion are most suggestive of dissociative fugue. Because of the generalized nature of his amnesia and negative physical findings, substance-induced amnestic disorder an unlikely diagnosis. There is insufficient evidence of distinct alternative personalities to diagnose dissociative identity disorder.

Used with permission from Williams & Wilkins, *Board Review Series: Psychiatry*, 1997.

Adjustment Disorders

10

Definition. Maladaptive reactions to an identifiable psychosocial stressor

Risk Factors/Etiology. Cause: environmental stressors having an effect on functioning. Risk that a stressor will cause an adjustment disorder depends on an individual's emotional strength and coping skills.

Prevalence. Extremely common; all age groups

Onset. Within 3 months of the initial presence of the stressor.

Course. Lasts 6 months or less once the stressor is resolved. Can become chronic if stressor continues and new ways of coping with the stressor are not developed.

Key Symptoms. Complaints of overwhelming anxiety, depression, or emotional turmoil associated with specific stressors

Associated Problems. Social and occupational performance deteriorate, erratic or withdrawn behavior.

Treatment

- Remove or ameliorate the stressor.
- Brief psychotherapy to improve coping skills
- Pharmacotherapy: Anxiolytic or antidepressant medications are used to ameliorate symptoms if therapy is not effective.

Differential Diagnosis. Normal reaction to stress. Disorders that occur following stress (e.g., GAD, PTSD, major depressive disorder).

Types.

- Depressed mood
- Anxiety
- Mixed anxiety and depressed mood
- Disturbance of conduct
- Mixed disturbance of emotions and conduct

Review Question

A 28-year-old woman without previous behavioral problems becomes angry and bitter after her husband of 5 years leaves her to live with his female business partner. One week later, the woman quits her job without giving notice and begins drinking heavily. For the next several weeks, the woman telephones friends and tearfully expresses her feelings. She also makes several threatening calls to her husband's new girlfriend.

Which of the following is the most likely diagnosis?

(A)   Adjustment disorder

(B)   Alcohol-induced mood disorder

(C)   Bipolar I disorder

(D)   Bipolar II disorder

(E)   Borderline personality disorder

Answer: A. Depression and erratic behavior after an interpersonal stressor are most suggestive of adjustment disorder with mixed disturbance of emotions and conduct. The cause of the symptoms is most likely the stressor and not the physiologic result of alcohol. Bipolar disorders I and II are unlikely diagnoses for an individual who has no history of mood episodes. Borderline personality disorder is a less likely diagnosis for an individual who has no history of past behavioral and interpersonal difficulties.

Used with permission from Williams & Wilkins, *Board Review Series: Psychiatry*, 1997.

Substance-Related and Addictive Disorders

11

Definitions

- **Substance use disorder:** negative behavioral, cognitive, and/or physiologic symptoms due to use of a substance, yet use continues despite these adverse consequences
- **Intoxication:** reversible substance-specific syndrome due to recent use of a substance
- **Withdrawal:** substance-specific behavioral, cognitive, and/or physiologic change due to the cessation or reduction in heavy or prolonged substance use

Physical and Psychiatric Examination

- **Substance abuse history:** Includes the substance(s) used, dosage(s), effects, duration and social context of use, and prior experiences with substance detoxification, rehabilitation, and relapse prevention
- **Medical history:** Includes complications of substance abuse
- **Psychiatric history:** Includes other primary psychiatric diagnoses and past treatments
- **Mental status examination:** Includes signs of substance-induced disorders
- **Physical examination:** Includes signs of substance use

Risk Factors/Etiology

- **Family history:** Biological sons of alcoholics are more likely to develop alcoholism than is the general population.
- **Physiology:** Individuals who are innately more tolerant to alcohol may be more likely to develop alcohol abuse.
- **Developmental history:** Poor parenting, childhood physical or sexual abuse, and permissive attitudes toward drug use.
- **Environmental risk factors:** Exposure to drug use through peers or certain occupations, economic disadvantage, and social isolation.
- **Psychiatric disturbances:** Conduct disorder, ADHD, depression, and low self-esteem.
- **Self-medication hypotheses:** Individuals with certain psychologic problems may abuse substances in an effort to alleviate symptoms (e.g., a person suffering from an anxiety disorder uses alcohol to decrease innate anxiety).

Diagnostic Tests

CAGE. Affirmative answers to any 2 of the following questions (or to the last question alone) are suggestive of alcohol abuse:

- Have you ever felt that you should cut down your drinking?
- Have you ever felt annoyed by others who have criticized your drinking?
- Have you ever felt guilty about your drinking?
- Have you ever had a morning drink (eye-opener) to steady your nerves or alleviate a hangover?

Urine drug screen: typically tests for amphetamines, barbiturates, benzodiazepines, cannabinoids, cocaine, methodone, methaqualone, opiates, phencyclidine

Hair testing: typically tests for cocaine, amphetamines, methamphetamines, opiates, PCP, marijuana

Breath: typically tests for alcohol

Blood: increased AST, ALT, and GGT for alcohol abuse

Types of treatment.

- **Pharmacotherapy:** medications that work on the reward center, such as naltrexone, varenicline, and bupropion.
- **Psychotherapy:** preferably group therapy such as Alcoholics Anonymous, Narcotics Anonymous
- **Behavioral modification** techniques: disulfiram (aversive conditioning), patch, gum, inhaler (fading)
- **Detoxification units:** typically 5-10 days, provide medications to assure safe withdrawal from substances
- **Rehabilitation programs:** typically 28-day programs, learn about relapse prevention and identification of triggers

Table I-11-1. Blood Alcohol Levels and Effects on Behavior

Blood Alcohol Level	Behavioral Effect
0.05%	Thought, judgment, and restraint are loosened and disrupted
0.1%	Motor actions become clumsy
0.2%	• Motor area of the brain is depressed • Emotional behavior is affected
0.3%	Confused or stuporous
0.4–0.5%	• Coma • At higher levels, death may occur due to respiratory depression

Table I-11-2. Substances of Abuse

Substance	Signs and Symptoms of Intoxication	Treatment of Intoxication	Signs and Symptoms of Withdrawal	Treatment of Withdrawal
Alcohol	Talkativeness, sullenness, gregariousness, moodiness, etc.	Mechanical ventilation, if severe	Tremors, hallucinations, seizures, delirium tremens	Benzodiazepines Thiamine Multivitamin Folic acid
Amphetamines, cocaine	Euphoria, hypervigilance, autonomic hyperactivity, weight loss, papillary dilatation, perceptual disturbances	Short-term use of antipsychotics, benzodiazepines, vitamin C to promote excretion in urine, anti-hypertensives	Anxiety, tremulousness, headache, increased appetite, depression, risk of suicide	Antidepressants
Anabolic steroids	Irritability, aggression, mood changes, psychosis, heart problems, liver problems, etc.	Symptomatic, abstinence	Depression, risk of suicide	SSRIs
Bath salts	Headache, palpitations, hallucinations, paranoia, violence, increased heart rate and blood pressure	Supportive, benzodiazepines	Unknown	Unknown
Benzodiazepines	Inappropriate sexual or aggressive behavior, impairment in memory or concentration	Flumazenil	Autonomic hyperactivity, tremors, insomnia, seizures, anxiety	Benzodiazepines
Cannabis	Impaired motor coordination, slowed sense of time, social withdrawal, conjunctival injection, increased appetite, dry mouth, tachycardia	None	None	None
Ecstasy	Euphoria, mild psychedelia, hyponatremia, seizures, death, rhabdomyolisis, increased heart rate, blood pressure, and temperature	Cyproheptadine, benzodiazepines, dantrolene	Unknown	Unknown
Hallucinogens	Ideas of reference, perceptual disturbances, impaired judgment, dissociative symptoms, pupillary dilatation, tremors, incoordination	Supportive counseling (talking down), antipsychotics, benzodiazepines	None	None

(Continued)

Table I-12-2. Substances of Abuse (*Cont'd*)

Substance	Signs and Symptoms of Intoxication	Treatment of Intoxication	Signs and Symptoms of Withdrawal	Treatment of Withdrawal
Inhalants	Belligerence, apathy, assaultiveness, impaired judgment, blurred vision, stupor or coma	Antipsychotics if delirious or agitated	None	None
Opiates	Apathy, dysphoria, papillary constriction, drowsiness, slurred speech, impairment in memory, coma or death	Naloxone	Fever, chills, lacrimation, runny nose, abdominal cramps, muscle spasms, insomnia, yawning	Clonidine, methadone
Phencyclidine (PCP)	Belligerence, assaultiveness, psychomotor agitation, nystagmus, hypertension, seizures, coma, hyperacusis	Talking down, benzodiazepines, antipsychotics	None	None

---

Review Question

A 29-year-old man is brought in by judicial order for evaluation of his continued involvement with heroin use. The man denies that he is addicted but is willing to enter treatment to avoid more severe criminal penalties.

Which of the following is essential to determine the presence of heroin use disorder in this individual?

(A)   A family history of substance abuse

(B)   Numerous arrests for dealing heroin

(C)   He vehemently denies that his use of heroin causes him any problems

(D)   He spends all his time trying to obtain heroin and can't stop himself from using it

(E)   He is not cooperative with treatment planning

Answer: D. Substance use disorder is characterized by the presence of a constellation of symptoms that suggest compulsive substance use, monopolization of time by substance-related activities, social and occupational consequences, and physiologic changes including tolerance and withdrawal. A family history of substance abuse, arrests for drug dealing, denial of substance-related problems, and cooperation with treatment may all occur in individuals with substance dependence, but are not diagnostic when occurring by themselves.

Used with permission from Williams & Wilkins, *Board Review Series: Psychiatry*, 1997.

Impulse Control Disorders 12

In impulse control disorders, patients are unable to resist a negative impulse. Before the act they have increased anxiety and after the act they feel a reduction in anxiety. Impulse control is mediated by the serotonergic system.

INTERMITTENT EXPLOSIVE DISORDER

> The police recently arrested a 24-year-old man after he beat up an older man, causing severe injury to his head and neck area and requiring more than 100 stitches. When asked why he assaulted the older man, he replied, "He took my potato chips."

Definition. A disorder characterized by discrete episodes of failure to resist aggressive impulses that result in serious assaultive acts or destruction of property. The degree of the aggressive act is typically out of proportion to the stressor. The attacks may occur within minutes or hours and tend to resolve spontaneously.

Risk Factors/Epidemiology. Affects men more than women, especially men in prisons and women in psychiatric facilities. May have genetic linkage because it is seen frequently among first-degree relatives. Patients may have had a history of head trauma, seizures, encephalitis, hyperactivity, or other brain dysfunctions. May be linked to low levels of 5HIAA, abnormalities in the limbic system, or testosterone. The symptoms lessen as the patients age.

Physical and Psychiatric Presenting Symptoms
- Neurologic examination may reveal soft signs, such as right–left ambivalence
- EEG usually normal
- Psychologic tests often normal
- Poor work histories
- Marital difficulties
- Problems with the law

Treatment. Pharmacotherapy consisting of anticonvulsants, antipsychotics, beta-blockers, or SSRIs has been somewhat helpful. Psychotherapy, although not the preferred treatment, may be beneficial. When psychotherapy is used, it must be with pharmacotherapy and in a group setting.

Differential Diagnosis
- *Medical:* Epilepsy, brain tumors, degenerative disease, and endocrine disorders
- *Psychiatric:* Antisocial personality disorder, borderline personality disorder, schizophrenia, and substance intoxication

KLEPTOMANIA

> A 25-year-old woman has a history of more than 20 arrests for stealing small items. She comes from a wealthy family and her parents do not understand her behavior. At home she has numerous salt and pepper shakers, napkin rings, and ashtrays, none of which she needs.

Definition. A disorder characterized by the recurrent failure to resist impulses to steal objects that the patient does not need. There is increased anxiety prior to the act, followed by release of anxiety after the act. The act of stealing is the goal.

Risk Factors/Epidemiology. Appears to be more common in women. Symptoms may be linked to stress in the patient's life. Often associated with mood disorders, OCDs, and eating disorders, such as bulimia nervosa. It has been linked to brain disease and ID.

Physical and Psychiatric Presenting Symptoms. May have signs of anxiety and depression. Feel guilty or ashamed of their actions.

Treatment. Insight-oriented therapy may be indicated to help the patients understand their behavior. Behavioral therapy, including aversive conditioning and systematic desensitization, has been helpful in some patients. If pharmacotherapy is indicated, consider SSRIs or anticonvulsants.

Differential Diagnosis

- *Medical:* None
- *Psychiatric:* Antisocial personality disorder, malingering, mania, and schizophrenia

PYROMANIA

> A 19-year-old teen with mild ID is arrested after he is found setting the neighbor's garbage cans on fire. Neighbors had observed him in the past starting fires in his own backyard, staring at them for hours, watching them burn.

Definition. A disorder characterized by deliberate fire-setting on more than one occasion. There is anxiety before the act and a release of anxiety after the act, sometimes followed by fascination and gratification. Must rule out arson.

Risk Factors/Epidemiology. Seen more frequently in men who are mildly retarded and may have a history of alcohol abuse. Many have histories of truancy and cruelty to animals.

Physical and Psychiatric Presenting Symptoms. Many watch fires in their neighborhoods and/ or set off fire alarms. Lack remorse for the consequences of their actions, and show resentment toward authority figures. May become sexually aroused by the fire.

Treatment. Because no treatment has been proven to be beneficial, incarceration may be indicated.

Differential Diagnosis

- *Medical:* Brain dysfunctions
- *Psychiatric:* Antisocial personality disorder, conduct disorder, mania, and schizophrenia

GAMBLING DISORDER

A 40-year-old married man and father of two, was fired from his job because of embezzlement of company funds, which he used to gamble with. When found, he did not have the money on him and admitted to losing it at a casino. His wife left him two months ago, and he has not seen his wife or children since then.

In DSM-5, this is now included under Substance-related and Addictive Disorders.

Definition. A disorder characterized by persistent and recurrent gambling behavior that includes a preoccupation with gambling, a need to gamble with more money, attempts to stop gambling and/or to win back losses, illegal acts to finance the gambling, or loss of relationships due to gambling.

Risk Factors/Epidemiology. More common in men, and seen in their parents as well. Increased incidence of alcohol dependence. May be predisposed by death, loss of a loved one, poor parenting, exposure to gambling behavior, and/or divorce. May be linked to mood disorders, OCDs, panic disorder, agoraphobia, and ADHD.

Physical and Psychiatric Presenting Symptoms

- May engage in antisocial behavior to obtain money for gambling
- Appear overconfident
- Suicide attempts
- Multiple arrests and/or incarceration

Treatment. Gamblers anonymous (GA) is the most effective treatment. It involves public confessions, peer pressure, and sponsors. Although pharmacotherapy is usually not indicated, some studies have shown some efficacy with SSRIs.

Differential Diagnosis

- *Medical:* None
- *Psychiatric:* Mania, antisocial personality disorder

TRICHOTILLOMANIA

A 20-year-old woman is rushed to the hospital after she complains of severe abdominal pain. She appears thin and withdrawn and is missing a lot of hair from both her scalp and eyebrows. A physical examination reveals an intestinal obstruction.

In DSM-5, this is now included under Obsessive-Compulsive and Related Disorders.

Definition. A disorder characterized by pulling one's own hair, resulting in hair loss. There is anxiety before the act and a release of anxiety after the act.

Risk Factors/Epidemiology. Affects women more than men. Associated disorders include OCD, obsessive-compulsive personality disorder, and depressive disorders.

Physical and Psychiatric Presenting Symptoms

- Hair loss is significant over all areas of the body.
- Area most affected is the scalp.
- May eat the hair, resulting in bezoars, obstruction, and malnutrition
- Head-banging, nail-biting, and gnawing may be present.
- Examination of the scalp reveals short, broken hairs along with long hairs.

Treatment. Treatment usually consists of behavior-modification techniques to decrease patient's anxiety; as well as pharmacotherapy, such as SSRIs, anticonvulsants, or antipsychotics to help decrease the urges.

Differential Diagnosis

- *Medical:* Alopecia areata, tinea capitis (biopsy would be indicated)
- *Psychiatric:* OCD, factitious disorder

Review Question

A 22-year-old woman was recently seen at her college graduation hoarding food in her purse and briefcase. When asked why, she replied, "I might be hungry later." She appeared to be of average height and weight, but with poor dentition. She has numerous calluses on the backs of both hands.

Which of the following disorders is she at risk for developing?

(A) Trichotillomania

(B) Kleptomania

(C) Gambling disorder

(D) Pyromania

(E) Intermittent explosive disorder

Answer: B. Patients with bulimia nervosa have an increased incidence of kleptomania. These patients will steal things they do not need.

ANOREXIA NERVOSA

Definition. Characterized by failure to maintain a normal body weight, fear and preoccupation with gaining weight and unrealistic self-evaluation as overweight. Subtypes are restricting (no binge-eating or purging) and binge-eating/purging (regularly engaged in binge-eating/purging).

Risk Factors/Etiology. Biologic factors are suggested by higher concordance for illness in monozygotic twins and the fact that amenorrhea may precede abnormal eating behavior. Psychologic risk factors include emotional conflicts concerning family control and sexuality. A cultural risk factor may be an emphasis on thinness.

Prevalence. 0.5%. Occurs at a 1:10 male-to-female ratio.

Onset. Average age is 17 years. Very late–onset anorexia nervosa has a poorer prognosis. Onset is often associated with emotional stressors, particularly conflicts with parents about independence, and sexual conflicts.

Key Symptoms

- Restricted food intake and maintaining diets of low-calorie foods. Weight loss may also be achieved through purging (i.e., vomiting or taking laxatives, diuretics, or enemas) and exercise.
- Great concern with appearance. Significant amount of time spent examining and denigrating self for perceived signs of excess weight.
- Denial of emaciated conditions
- With binge-eating/purging: Self-induced vomiting; laxative and diuretic abuse

Associated Symptoms. Excessive interest in food-related activities (other than eating), obsessive-compulsive symptoms, depressive symptoms.

Course. Some individuals recover after a single episode, and others develop a waxing-and-waning course.

Outcome. Long-term mortality rate of individuals hospitalized for anorexia nervosa is 10%, resulting from the effects of starvation and purging or suicide.

Physical Examination. Signs of malnutrition include emaciation, hypotension, bradycardia, lanugo (i.e., fine hair on the trunk), and peripheral edema. Signs of purging include eroded dental enamel caused by emesis and scarred or scratched hands from self-gagging to induce emesis. There may be evidence of general medical conditions caused by abnormal diets, starvation, and purging.

Diagnostic Tests

- **Signs of malnutrition:** normochromic, normocytic anemia, elevated liver enzymes, abnormal electrolytes, low estrogen and testosterone levels, sinus bradycardia, reduced brain mass, and abnormal EEG
- **Signs of purging:** metabolic alkalosis, hypochloremia, and hypokalemia caused by emesis; metabolic acidosis caused by laxative abuse

Treatment. Initial treatment should be correction of significant physiologic consequences of starvation with hospitalization if necessary. Behavioral therapy should be initiated, with rewards or punishments based on absolute weight, not on eating behaviors. Family therapy designed to reduce conflicts about control by parents is often helpful. Antidepressants may play a limited role in treatment when comorbid depression is present.

Differential Diagnosis. Major rule-outs are bulimia nervosa, general medical conditions that cause weight loss, major depressive disorder, schizophrenia, OCD, and body dysmorphic disorder.

BULIMIA NERVOSA AND BINGE EATING DISORDER

Definition. Characterized by frequent binge-eating and a self-image that is unduly influenced by weight. Types:

- **Bulimia nervosa:** binge-eating and purging behavior
- **Binge-eating disorder:** binge-eating but no purging behavior

Risk Factors/Etiology. Psychologic conflict regarding guilt, helplessness, self-control, and body image may predispose. Biologic factors are suggested by frequent association with mood disorders.

Prevalence. 2% in young adult females. Occurs at a 1:9 male-to-female ratio

Onset. Usually during late adolescence or early adulthood and often follows a period of dieting

Course. May be chronic or intermittent

Outcome. 70% of cases have remitted after 10 years. Co-occurring substance abuse is associated with a poorer prognosis

Key Symptoms

- **Recurrent episodes of binge-eating in both binge-eating disorder and bulemia.** Obsession with dieting but followed by binge-eating of high-calorie foods. Binges are associated with emotional stress and followed by feelings of guilt, self-recrimination, and compensatory behaviors.
- **Recurrent, inappropriate compensatory behavior in bulemia but not in binge-eating disorder.** After a binge, attempts to prevent weight gain through self-induced vomiting, misuse of laxatives, diuretics, enemas, or other medications; fasting; or excessive exercise.
- **Self-evaluation is unduly influenced by body shape and weight in bulemia.** Self-castigation for mild weight gain or binges. Attempts to conceal binge-eating or purging, or lies about behaviors.

Associated Problems. Depressive symptoms, substance abuse, and impulsivity (e.g., kleptomania)

Comorbid Disorders. Borderline personality disorder present in about 50%

Physical Examination. Evidence of purging

Diagnostic Tests. Evidence of laxative or diuretic abuse

Treatment. Cognitive and behavioral therapy are major treatment. Psychodynamic psychotherapies are useful for accompanying borderline personality traits. Antidepressant medications, particularly SSRIs, are usually employed.

Differential Diagnosis. Major rule-outs are anorexia nervosa, binge-eating/purging, major depressive disorder with atypical features, and borderline personality disorder.

Review Question

A 19-year-old woman is hospitalized for dehydration caused by severe, laxative-induced diarrhea. She is depressed about the recent breakup of a romantic relationship. She admits that she uses laxatives because she has been binge-eating frequently and is worried about gaining weight. Although the woman has BMI 16, she believes that she is overweight.

Which of the following is the most likely diagnosis?

(A)   Anorexia nervosa

(B)   Brief psychotic disorder

(C)   Bulimia nervosa

(D)   Delusional disorder, somatic type

(E)   Major depressive disorder

Answer: A. The patient presents with low body weight, a distorted body image, a fear of obesity, and amenorrhea, all of which strongly suggest anorexia nervosa. Bingeing and purging behavior is commonly present with this disorder. Because this individual has the essential features of anorexia nervosa, the diagnosis of bulimia nervosa is not made. Because the woman shows no evidence of delusions, brief psychotic disorder or delusional disorder are unlikely diagnoses. Although depression commonly accompanies eating disorders, it does not appear to be the primary problem in this woman's case.

Used with permission from Williams & Wilkins, *Board Review Series: Psychiatry*, 1997.

Personality Disorders 14

Definition. Characterized by personality patterns that are pervasive, inflexible, and maladaptive. There are 3 clusters:

Cluster A: Peculiar thought processes, inappropriate affect

Cluster B: Mood lability, dissociative symptoms, preoccupation with rejection

Cluster C: Anxiety, preoccupation with criticism or rigidity

Risk Factors/Etiology. Personality disorders (PDs) are the product of the interaction of inborn temperament and subsequent developmental environment. Risk factors include innate temperamental difficulties, such as irritability; adverse environmental events, such as child neglect or abuse; and personality disorders in parents.

Prevalence. All are relatively common. More males have antisocial and narcissistic PDs, more females have borderline and histrionic PDs.

Onset. Usually not diagnosed until late adolescence or early adulthood

Course. Usually very chronic over decades without treatment. Symptoms of paranoid, schizoid, and narcissistic PD often worsen with age; symptoms of antisocial and borderline PD often ameliorate.

Key Symptoms. Long pattern of difficult interpersonal relationships, problems adapting to stress, failure to achieve goals, chronic unhappiness, low self-esteem

Associated Diagnoses. Mood disorders

Treatment. Psychotherapy is the mainstay of treatment. Intensive and long-term psychodynamic and cognitive therapy are treatments of choice for most PDs. Use of mood stabilizers and antidepressants is sometimes useful for Cluster B PDs.

Differential Diagnosis. Major rule-outs are mood disorders, personality change due to a general medical condition, and adjustment disorders.

SPECIFIC PERSONALITY DISORDERS

Cluster A

Paranoid PD: Distrust and suspiciousness. Individuals are mistrustful and suspicious of the motivations and actions of others and are often secretive and isolated. They are emotionally cold and odd.

A 57-year-old man living in a condominium complex constantly accuses his neighbors of plotting to avoid payment of their share of maintenance. He writes angry letters to other owners and has initiated several lawsuits. He lives alone and does not socialize.

Schizoid PD: Detachment and restricted emotionality. Individuals are emotionally distant. They are disinterested in others and indifferent to praise or criticism. Associated features include social drifting and dysphoria.

A 24-year-old man lives alone and works nights as a security guard. He ignores invitations from coworkers to socialize and has no outside interests.

Schizotypal PD: Discomfort with social relationships; thought distortion; eccentricity. Individuals are socially isolated and uncomfortable with others. Unlike Schizoid PD, they have peculiar patterns of thinking, including ideas of reference and persecution, odd preoccupations, and odd speech and affect. DSM-5 includes this PD in both psychotic disorders and personality disorders.

A 30-year-old man is completely preoccupied with the study and the brewing of herbal teas. He associates many peculiar powers with such infusions and says that plants bring him extra luck. He spends all of his time alone, often taking solitary walks in the wilderness for days at a time, collecting plants for teas. He has no history of disorganized behavior. At times he believes that songs on the radio are about his life.

Cluster B

Histrionic PD. Usually characterized by colorful, exaggerated behavior and excitable, shallow expression of emotions; uses physical appearance to draw attention to self; sexually seductive; and is uncomfortable in situations where he or she is not the center of attention.

A 30-year-old woman presents to the doctor's office dressed in a sexually seductive manner and insists that the doctor comment on her appearance. When the doctor refuses to do so, she becomes upset.

Borderline PD. Usually characterized by an unstable affect, mood swings, marked impulsivity, unstable relationships, recurrent suicidal behaviors, chronic feelings of emptiness or boredom, identity disturbance, and inappropriate anger. If stressed, may become psychotic. Main defense mechanism is splitting.

A 20-year-old nurse was recently admitted after reporting auditory hallucinations, which have occurred during the last few days. She reports marriage difficulties and believes her husband is to blame for the problem. She has several scars on her wrists and has a history of substance abuse.

Antisocial PD. Usually characterized by continuous antisocial or criminal acts, inability to conform to social rules, impulsivity, disregard for the rights of others, aggressiveness, lack of remorse, and deceitfulness. These have occurred since the age of 15, and the individual is at least 18 years of age.

> A 22-year-old man was recently arrested after he set his mother's house on fire. He has had numerous problems with the law, which started at an early age when he was sent to a juvenile detention center for his behavior at both home and school. He lacks remorse for setting the fire and expresses a desire that his mother would have died in the fire.

Narcissistic PD. Usually characterized by a sense of self-importance, grandiosity, and preoccupation with fantasies of success. This person believes s/he is special, requires excessive admiration, reacts with rage when criticized, lacks empathy, is envious of others, and is interpersonally exploitative.

> A famous actor is outraged when a director questions his acting abilities during rehearsal for a play. The actor responds by walking off the stage and not returning to the stage unless the director apologizes publicly for her behavior.

Cluster C

Avoidant PD. Individuals have social inhibition, feelings of inadequacy, and hypersensitivity to criticism. They shy away from work or social relationships because of fears of rejection that are based on feelings of inadequacy. They feel lonely and substandard and are preoccupied with rejection.

> A 43-year-old man dreads an upcoming company holiday party because he believes that he is incapable of engaging in social conversation or dancing. He believes that he will become an object of pity or ridicule if he attempts such things. He anticipates yet another lonely holiday.

Dependent PD: Submissive and clinging behavior related to a need to be taken care of. Individuals are consumed with the need to be taken care of. They have clinging behavior and worry unrealistically about abandonment. They feel inadequate and helpless and avoid disagreements with others. They usually focus dependency on a family member or spouse and desperately seek a substitute should this person become unavailable. Associated features include self-doubt, excessive humility, poor independent functioning, mood disorders, anxiety disorders, adjustment disorder, and other PDs.

> A 26-year-old man is brought into the emergency room after sustaining severe rectal lacerations during a sadistic sexual episode with his partner. The patient is extremely concerned that the police not be informed because he doesn't want to upset his partner and cause the partner to leave.

Obsessive-Compulsive PD. Individuals are preoccupied with orderliness, perfectionism, and control. They are often consumed by the details of everything and lose their sense of over-all goals. They are strict and perfectionistic, overconscientious, and inflexible. They may be obsessed with work and productivity and are hesitant to delegate tasks to others. Other traits include being miserly and unable to give up possessions. This PD should not be confused with OCD, a separate disorder. Associated features include indecisiveness, dysphoria, anger, social inhibition, and difficult interpersonal relationships.

> A 37-year-old woman seeks psychotherapy as a result of an impending divorce. She states that her demands to keep the house spotless, to maintain an extremely detailed and fixed work and recreational schedule, and to observe rigid dietary habits have driven her spouse away.

Normal Sleep and Sleep Disorders 15

NORMAL SLEEP

Sleep Stages

Sleep is divided into 2 stages, nonrapid eye movement (NREM) and rapid eye movement (REM). There are numerous differences between them.

NREM. A state of sleep characterized by slowing of the EEG rhythms, high muscle tone, absence of eye movements, and thoughtlike mental activity. In this state the brain is inactive while the body is active. NREM is made up of 4 stages:

Table I-15-1. NREM

Stage	EEG Findings	Distribution
Stage 1	Disappearance of alpha wave and appearance of theta wave	5%
Stage 2	k complexes and sleep spindles	45%
Stage 3	Appearance of delta wave	12%
Stage 4	Continuation of delta wave	13%

REM (Rapid Eye Movement). A stage of sleep characterized by aroused EEG patterns, sexual arousal, saccadic eye movements, generalized muscular atony (except middle-ear and eye muscles), and dreams. In this state, the brain is active and the body is inactive.

Table I-15-2. REM

Stage	EEG Findings	Distribution
REM	Bursts of sawtooth waves	25%

Sleep Facts

Table I-15-3. Sleep Facts (Stage 2–REM)

Stage	Fact(s)
Stage 2	Longest of all the sleep stages
Stages 3 and 4	Also called slow wave or delta sleep Hardest to arouse Tends to vanish in the elderly
REM	Easiest to arouse Lengthens in time as night progresses Increased during the second half of the night

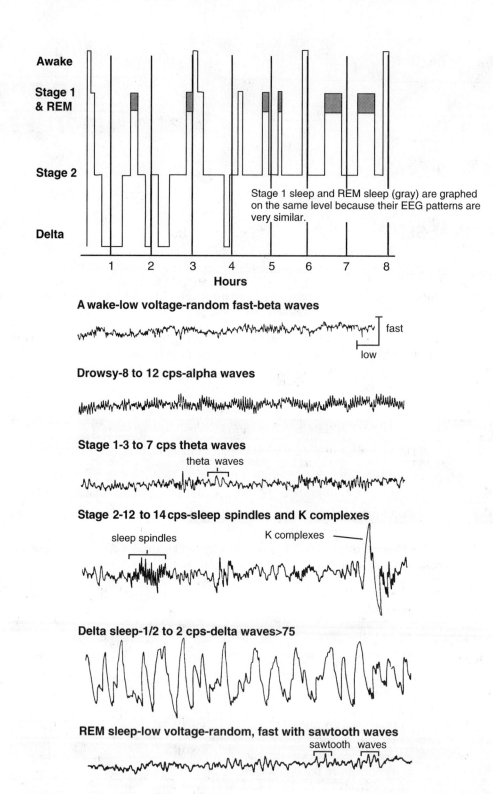

Stage 1 sleep and REM sleep (gray) are graphed on the same level because their EEG patterns are very similar.

Figure I-15-1. Sleep Architecture Diagram Showing Stages of Sleep in Sequence

Sleep Latency. The time needed before you actually fall asleep. Typically less than 15 minutes in most individuals; however, may be abnormal in many disorders, such as insomnia, etc.

REM Latency. The period lasting from the moment you fall asleep to the first REM period. Lasts approximately 90 minutes in most individuals. However, several disorders will shorten REM latency; these disorders include depression and narcolepsy.

Characteristics of Sleep from Infancy to Old Age

- Total sleep time decreases.
- REM percentage decreases.
- Stages 3 and 4 tend to vanish.

Neurotransmitters of Sleep

- **Serotonin:** Increased during sleep; initiates sleep
- **Acetylcholine:** Increased during sleep; linked to REM sleep
- **Norepinephrine:** Decreased during sleep; linked to REM sleep
- **Dopamine:** Increased toward end of sleep; linked to arousal and wakefulness

Chemical Effects on Sleep

- **Tryptophan:** Increases total sleep time
- **Dopamine agonists:** Produce arousal
- **Dopamine antagonists:** Decrease arousal, thus produce sleep
- **Benzodiazepines:** Suppress Stage 4 and, when used chronically, increase sleep latency
- **Alcohol intoxication:** Suppresses REM
- **Barbiturate intoxication:** Suppresses REM
- **Alcohol withdrawal:** REM rebound
- **Barbiturate withdrawal:** REM rebound
- **Major depression:** Shortened REM latency, increased REM time, suppression of delta, multiple awakenings, and early morning awakening

SLEEP DISORDERS

Narcolepsy

A 35-year-old man was recently hospitalized for the tenth time after he crashed his car into a post. When questioned, he did not remember the cause of the accident and had just had his license suspended. His friends reported occasions when he fell asleep during dinner and during conversations with them.

Definition. A disorder characterized by excessive daytime sleepiness and abnormalities of REM sleep for a period of greater than 3 months. REM sleep occurs in less than 10 minutes. Patients feel refreshed upon awakening.

Physical and Psychiatric Presenting Symptoms

- **Sleep attacks:** Most common symptom
- **Cataplexy:** Pathognomonic sign, consisting of a sudden loss of muscle tone which may have been precipitated by a loud noise or intense emotion. If short episode, the patient remains awake.
- **Hypnagogic and hypnopompic hallucinations:** Hallucinations that occur as the patient is going to sleep and is waking up from sleep, respectively.
- **Sleep paralysis:** Most often occurs during awakening, when the patient is awake but unable to move.
- Report falling asleep quickly at night

Treatment. Forced naps at a regular time of day is usually the treatment of choice. When medications are given, psychostimulants are preferred. If cataplexy is present, antidepressants such as TCAs are preferred. Gamma-hydroxybutyrate (GHB) is also used for narcolepsy–cataplexy by improving the quality of nighttime sleep.

Sleep Apnea

An overweight man reports having difficulties in his marriage because of his snoring at night. During the day, he reports feeling tired despite sleeping for 8 hours at night.

Definition. A disorder characterized by the cessation of airflow at the nose or mouth during sleep. These apneic episodes usually last longer than 10 seconds each. Characterized by a loud snore followed by a heavy pause. Considered pathologic if the patient has more than 5 episodes an hour or more than 30 episodes during the night. In severe cases, patients may experience more than 300 apneic episodes during the night.

Physical and Psychiatric Presenting Symptoms

- Usually seen in obese, middle-aged males
- Sometimes associated with depression, mood changes, and daytime sleepiness
- Spouses typically complain of partner's snoring, and of partner's restlessness during the night
- Complain of dry mouth in the morning
- May have headaches in the morning
- Complain of being tired during the day
- May develop arrhythmias, hypoxemia, pulmonary hypertension, and sudden death

Types of Sleep Apnea

- *Obstructive:* Muscle atonia in oropharynx; nasal, tongue, or tonsil obstruction
- *Central:* Lack of respiratory effort
- *Mixed:* Central at first, but prolonged due to collapse of the airway

Treatment. Continuous positive nasal airway pressure is the treatment of choice. Other treatment includes weight loss, surgery. Sleeping on one's side instead of one's back will help keep the airways open.

Insomnia

While studying over the past week for an important exam, Michael, a third-year medical student, has been unable to sleep for the past several days. At night, he lies awake and imagines himself doing poorly on the exam and failing medical school. During the day, he is tired and frequently falls asleep during his classes.

Definition. A disorder characterized by difficulties in initiating or maintaining sleep.

Risk Factors/Epidemiology. Typically associated with some form of anxiety or anticipatory anxiety. Many patients have underlying psychiatric disorders, such as depression, etc. If due to a psychiatric disorder, seen more frequently in women. Other conditions include PTSD, OCD, and eating disorders.

Physical and Psychiatric Presenting Symptoms

- Predominant complaint is difficulty initiating or maintaining sleep
- Affects the patient's level of functioning
- Frequent yawning and tiredness during the day

Treatment. Consider good sleep hygiene techniques, such as arising at same time of the day, avoiding daytime naps, avoiding evening stimulation, discontinuing CNS-acting drugs, taking hot baths near bedtime, eating meals at regular times, using relaxation techniques and maintaining comfortable sleeping conditions. If these do not work, consider behavioral modification techniques such as stimulus control. If medications are to be used, consider zolpidem, eszopiclone, or zaleplon.

Differential Diagnosis

- *Medical:* Pain, CNS lesions, endocrine diseases, aging, brain-stem lesions, alcohol, diet, medications
- *Psychiatric:* Anxiety, tension, depression, and environmental changes, other sleep disorders

Parasomnias

Table I-15-4. Parasomnias

Disorder	Sleep Stage	Characteristics	Treatment
Nightmares (dream anxiety disorder)	REM	• Memory of the event upon awakening • Increases during times of stress • Reported by 50% of the population	• Usually none indicated, but may use REM suppressants such as TCAs
Night terror (sleep terror disorder)	Stages 3 and 4	• Awakened by scream or intense anxiety • No memory of the event the following day • Seen more frequently in children • More common in boys • Runs in families	• Treatment rarely required • If medication is needed, consider benzodiazepines
Sleeptalking	All stages of sleep	• Common in children • Usually involves a few words • May accompany night terrors and sleepwalking	• No treatment is necessary
Sleepwalking	Stage 3 and 4	• Sequence of behaviors without full consciousness • May perform perseverative behaviors • Usually terminates in awakening followed by confusion • May return to sleep without any memory of the event • Begins at a young age • More common in boys • May find neurologic condition • Sleep deprivation may exacerbate	• Need to assure patient safety • Use drugs to suppress Stages 3 and 4, such as benzodiazepines

Review Questions

1. An overweight man of average height presents to his doctor's office complaining of feeling tired during the day. He has missed several days of work due to this problem. Which of the following is the most likely diagnosis?

   (A) Narcolepsy

   (B) Insomnia

   (C) Sleep apnea

   (D) Normal sleep pattern

   (E) Hypersomnia

2. Which of the following is the most likely explanation for a young man suddenly falling down but not losing consciousness?

   (A) Syncope

   (B) Cataplexy

   (C) Sleep paralysis

   (D) Medication toxicity

   (E) Hypotensive episode

3. Which of the following is the treatment of choice for insomnia?

   (A) Long-term use of benzodiazepines

   (B) Behavioral techniques

   (C) Drinking coffee before bedtime

   (D) Regular exercises before bedtime

   (E) Frequent naps during the day

1. **Answer: C.** Patients with sleep apnea have multiple episodes of waking up in the middle of the night. Therefore, they are tired during the day. These patients are typically unaware that they wake in the middle of the night.

2. **Answer: B.** Cataplexy is the sudden loss of muscle tone without loss of consciousness. It is differentiated from syncope in that syncope typically includes loss of consciousness. Patients with narcolepsy are usually young and do not have any blood pressure abnormalities.

3. **Answer: B.** Although benzodiazepines are regularly used for the treatment of insomnia, the best treatment includes behavioral techniques such as stimulus control. The patient leaves the bed whenever he is unable to fall asleep, therefore conditioning himself that the bed is only used for sleeping. Choices C, D, and E will tend to cause insomnia.

Sexual Identity. Based on the person's sexual characteristics, such as external and internal genitalia, hormonal characteristics, and secondary sexual characteristics

Gender Identity. Based on the person's sense of maleness or femaleness, established by age 3

Gender Role. Based on the external behavioral patterns that reflect the person's inner sense of gender identity

Sexual Orientation. Based on the person's choice of a love object; may be heterosexual (opposite sex), homosexual (same sex), bisexual (both sexes), or asexual (no sex)

MASTURBATION

- Normal precursor of object-related sexual behavior
- All men and women masturbate.
- Genital self-stimulation begins in early childhood
- As puberty arrives, sexual interest peaks and masturbation increases.
- Adolescents and adults typically have sexual fantasies while masturbating.
- Commonly seen among adolescents, married couples, and the elderly
- Excessive only if it interferes with daily functioning

HOMOSEXUALITY

- Removed from the DSM in 1980 as a mental illness
- Considered a variant of human sexuality, not a pathologic disorder
- Most homosexuals report feelings toward same sex individuals since adolescence.
- Recent studies indicate it may be due to genetic and biologic causes.
- Greater incidence among monozygotic versus dizygotic twins
- No difference in the sexual practices from those exhibited by heterosexuals.
- Male–male relationships may be less stable than female–female relationships.
- Equal incidence of mental illness when compared with heterosexuals.
- Exceptions (normal during adolescence):
  - Visual comparison of genitalia
  - Mutual masturbation
  - Group exhibitionism
  - Handholding, kissing, etc.

SEXUAL DYSFUNCTIONS

A group of disorders related to a particular phase of the sexual response cycle. These disorders can be psychologic, biologic, or both, and include, desire, arousal, orgasm, and pain.

Table I-16-1. Sexual Dysfunctions

Phase	Characteristics	Disorder	Treatment
Desire	Focuses on the patient's drives, motivation, and desires	**Hypoactive sexual desire:** patients have a decrease or absence of sexual fantasies, desires, etc. **Sexual aversion:** a complete aversion to all sexual contact	Address issues with patient, such as feelings of guilt, poor self-esteem, homosexual impulses, etc. Couples therapy may be indicated if due to marital conflict.
Arousal	Consists of a sense of sexual pleasure with accompanying physiologic changes	**Female sexual arousal:** persistent failure to achieve or maintain adequate lubrication during the sexual act **Impotence:** persistent or recurrent inability to attain or maintain adequate erection until completion of the sexual act	Address issues of guilt, anxiety, and fear. Evaluate for use of medications that cause vaginal dryness, such as antihistamines or anticholinergics. Instruct in relaxation techniques. Must rule out if organic versus psychological. Consider plethysmography or postage stamp test.
Orgasm	Physiologic state in which sexual tension is released and contractions are produced in various organs.	**Female orgasmic disorder and delayed ejaculation:** recurrent or persistent inability to achieve an orgasm either through masturbation or sexual intercourse **Premature ejaculation:** Ejaculation before the man wishes to do so, before penetration, or just after penetration	Address issues of guilt, fear of impregnation, etc. Treatment includes use of vibrators, education, and fantasy. Consider behavioral techniques such as squeeze and stop-and-go. Address issues of anxiety about the sexual act. Consider the use of SSRIs to delay ejaculation.
Pain	Subjective sense of pain associated with the sexual act. Most likely due to dynamic factors.	**Genito-pelvic pain disorder:** Pain associated with sexual intercourse in either male or female. Not diagnosed when organic cause has been found or if due to lack of vaginal lubrication. **Penetration disorder:** involuntary constriction of the outer one-third of the vagina that interferes with the sexual act	Help the woman deal with issues of anxiety and tension about the sexual act. Behavioral techniques, such as the use of dilators and relaxation. Address issues of fear of impregnation, strict upbringing, religion, etc.

PARAPHILIC DISORDER

A 20-year-old man was caught outside his neighbor's window, looking in as she disrobed. Before his arrest, he would wander the subway stations and rub himself up against women as well as expose himself to women who were nearby. All of these activities produced sexual pleasure in the patient.

Definition. A group of disorders that is recurrent and sexually arousing. Usually focus on humiliation and/or suffering and the use of nonliving objects and involve nonconsenting partners. Typically occur for >6 months and are usually distressing and cause impairment in patient's level of functioning.

Risk Factors/ Epidemiology. Affects men more than women. Peak incidence is age 15–25. Tend to have other paraphilias, and as the patient ages, the frequency decreases.

Physical and Psychiatric Presenting Symptoms

- Sexual activity is ritualistic.
- Fantasy is typically fixed and shows very little variation.
- Intense urge to carry out the fantasy

Treatment. Individual psychotherapy is indicated to help the patient understand the reasons why the paraphilia developed. Patient also becomes aware of daily activities and how they are related to the paraphilic behavior. Behavioral techniques, such as aversive conditioning, may be indicated in some situations. Pharmacotherapy consists of antiandrogens or SSRIs to help reduce patient's sexual drive.

Differential Diagnosis. Must distinguish between experimentation and actual paraphilias.

Types of Paraphilic Disorders

- **Exhibitionism:** recurrent urge to expose oneself to strangers
- **Fetishism:** involves the use of nonliving objects usually associated with the human body
- **Frotteurism:** recurrent urge or behavior involving touching or rubbing against a non-consenting partner
- **Pedophilia:** recurrent urges or arousal toward prepubescent children. Most common paraphilia.
- **Voyeurism:** recurrent urges or behaviors involving the act of observing an unsuspecting person who is engaging in sexual activity, disrobing, etc. Earliest paraphilia to develop.
- **Masochism:** recurrent urge or behavior involving the act of humiliation
- **Sadism:** recurrent urge or behavior involving acts in which physical or psychologic suffering of a victim is exciting to the patient.
- **Transvestic fetishism:** recurrent urge or behavior involving cross-dressing. Usually found in heterosexual men.

GENDER DYSPHORIA

Billy, a 5-year-old boy, was found in his parent's bedroom wearing his mother's clothes. He has been observed going to the bathroom to urinate while sitting on the toilet as well as playing with dolls instead of his trucks and guns. He prefers to wear dresses and hates being a boy.

Definition. Also called gender identity dysphoria. A disorder characterized by a persistent discomfort and sense of inappropriateness regarding the patient's assigned sex.

Risk Factors/Epidemiology. Seen more frequently in men than in women. Cause is unknown. Many believe it may be due to biologic reasons, such as hormones, etc.

Physical and Psychiatric Presenting Symptoms

- Children will have preference for friends of the opposite sex.
- Preoccupied with wearing opposite gender's clothes
- Refuse to urinate sitting down, if a girl, or standing up, if a boy
- Believe they were born with the wrong body
- Routinely request medications or surgery to change their physical appearance
- Women may bind their breasts, have mastectomies, take testosterone to deepen the voice.
- Men may have electrolysis to remove body hair and take estrogens to change the voice, and may have surgeries to remove the penis and create a vagina.

Review Questions

1. What is the treatment of choice for premature ejaculation?

   (A) Plethysmography
   (B) Dilators
   (C) Squeeze technique
   (D) Postage stamp
   (E) Aversive conditioning

2. What is the most common cause of erectile dysfunction due to a medical condition?

   (A) Pancreatitis
   (B) Diabetes
   (C) Cirrhosis
   (D) Myocardial infarction
   (E) UTI

---

1. **Answer: C.** The treatment of premature ejaculation typically consists of behavioral techniques aimed at prolonging the time before ejaculation occurs. These include the squeeze-and-go technique. Choices A and D are for the diagnosis of erectile dysfunction. Choice B is for the treatment of pain/penetration disorder.

2. **Answer: B.** Diabetes has been known to be a common cause of erectile dysfunction. Alcohol has been proven to be a common cause of erectile dysfunction in men of all ages.

Psychopharmacology 17

GENERAL PRINCIPLES OF ANTIPSYCHOTIC MEDICATION

Used to treat manifestations of psychosis and other psychiatric disorders.

Precise mechanism of antipsychotic action is unknown; however, antipsychotic medication (APM) blocks several populations of dopamine (D2, D4) receptors in the brain.

The newer antipsychotic medications also block some serotonin receptors (5HT), a property that may be associated with increased efficacy.

Antipsychotic medication also variably blocks central and peripheral cholinergic, histaminic, and alpha-adrenergic receptors.

Types of antipsychotic medications

- Typical: work mostly on dopamine receptors, treat the positive symptoms (hallucinations and delusions) and have many side effects (haloperidol, fluphenazine, chlorpromazine, etc.)
- Atypical: work mostly on dopamine and serotonin receptors, treat both positive and negative symptoms (flat affect, poor grooming, social withdrawal, anhedonia, etc), and have fewer side effects; always used as first-line agents (risperidone, olanzapine, etc.)

SIDE EFFECTS OF ANTIPSYCHOTIC MEDICATION

General

Sedation. Due to antihistaminic activity

Hypotension. Effect is due to alpha-adrenergic blockade and is most common with low-potency APMs.

Anticholinergic Symptoms. Dry mouth, blurred vision, urinary hesitancy, constipation, bradycardia, confusion, and delirium

Endocrine Effects. Gynecomastia, galactorrhea, and amenorrhea

Dermal and Ocular Syndromes. Photosensitivity, abnormal pigmentation, cataracts

Other Effects. Cardiac conduction abnormalities (especially with thioridazine), agranulocytosis with clozapine

Movement

Acute Dystonia. (Dystonic Reaction).

- Presentation: Spasms of various muscle groups
- Can be dramatic and frightening to patient
- Can be a major contributing factor to subsequent noncompliance with treatment
- Young men may be at higher risk, seen in 10% patients.
- Treatment: anticholinergics, such as benztropine, diphenhydramine, or trihexyphenidyl
- Can occur within hours after treatment

Akathisia

- Presenting Symptoms: Motor restlessness, "ants in your pants"
- Differential Diagnosis: Often mistaken for anxiety and agitation
- Treatment: lowering the dose, adding benzodiazepines or beta-blockers, switching to other antipsychotic medication
- Can occur several weeks after treatment

Tardive Dyskinesia (TD).

- Characterized by choreoathetosis and other involuntary movements
- Movements often occur first in the tongue or fingers and later involve the trunk.
- Etiology may be a form of "chemical denervation hypersensitivity," which is caused by chronic dopamine blockade in the basal ganglia.
- Patients who take high doses of older antipsychotic medication for long periods of time are at highest risk, and movements gradually worsen with continued use.
- Treatment: Use newer antipsychotic medications.
- Seen more frequently in elderly females
- Can occur after 3–6 months after treatment

Adverse Effects: Neuroleptic Malignant Syndrome

- Presentation: Fairly rare and potentially life-threatening condition characterized by muscular rigidity, hyperthermia, autonomic instability, and delirium. CPK will be elevated.
- Usually associated with high dosages of high-potency antipsychotic medication.
- Treatment: Immediate discontinuation of the medication and physiologic supportive measures; dantrolene or bromocriptine may be used.

ATYPICAL ANTIPSYCHOTIC MEDICATIONS

- Clozapine: gold standard for the treatment of schizophrenia; not used as first-line agent; may cause agranulocytosis (<1%) so monitoring of WBC is essential
- Risperidone: increased risk of movement disorders and elevation of prolactin
- Olanzapine: increased risk of weight gain, metabolic syndrome, diabetes, etc.
- Quetiapine: lowest risk of movement disorders
- Paliperidone: active metabolite of risperidone; fewer side effects than risperidone

- Ziprasidone: prolongation of Qt interval
- Aripiprazole: partial dopamine agonist at low doses, may be used as adjunct for depression
- Asenapine: sedation, akathisia
- Iloperidone: hypotension, dizziness, somnolence
- Lurasidone: somnolence, akathisia, weight gain

How to treat psychotic symptoms:

- First-line: always use atypical agents
- Emergency room: use short-acting intramuscular agent such as haloperidol, fluphenazine, olanzapine, or ziprasidone
- Non-adherant patient: use long-acting antipsychotic medication such as haloperidol, fluphenazine, risperidone, paliperidone, or olanzapine
- Last resort: clozapine
- All meds ineffective: may consider ECT

ANTIDEPRESSANT MEDICATIONS (ADs)

Clinical Guidelines

- Overall efficacy for treatment of major depressive disorder is around 70%.
- Newer ADs should be considered first because of better safety profile.
- Difficult to predict which patient will respond to which antidepressant, so trials of several antidepressants may be necessary before an effective one is found.
- Individual antidepressants differ greatly in their side-effect profiles and must be matched to patient preference and ability to tolerate.
- Older antidepressants are extremely dangerous when an overdose is ingested. When used to treat individuals with depressive symptoms, clinicians should generally prescribe in small quantities and only after determining the absence of suicidal intent.
- If no response to treatment after 4 weeks, or if patient cannot tolerate current antidepressant, switch to another.
- Treatment should continue for 6 months to 1 yr after favorable response.

Untoward Effects

- **Sedation:** due to histamine blockade
- **Hypotension:** due to alpha blockade
- **Anticholinergic effects:** dry mouth, blurry vision, urinary retention, confusion
- **Cardiac:** conduction abnormalities most marked with TCAs
- **Seizures:** bupropion (Wellbutrin)
- **Sexual dysfunction:** anorgasmia and decreased libido with SSRIs; priapism with trazodone (Desyrel)

SSRIs

Inhibit reuptake of serotonin

- **Types:** Fluoxetine (Prozac), paroxetine (Paxil), and sertraline (Zoloft), fluvoxamine. (Luvox), citalopram (Celexa), escitalopram (Lexapro)
- Reduced number of serious side effects
- Simple dosing schedules
- Significant incidence of agitation, nausea, vomiting, headache, diarrhea, and sexual dysfunction

Hybrid antidepressants (not real name)

- Venlafaxine: inhibit reuptake of NE and S, used for depression and anxiety, may cause hypertension, blurry vision, diaphoresis, etc.
- Desvenlafaxine: inhibit reuptake of NE and S, active metabolite of venlafaxine therefore fewer side effects
- Duloxetine: inhibit reuptake of NE and S, approved for depression and neuropathic pain
- Bupropion: inhibits reuptake of NE and dopamine, approved for depression and smoking cessation; may cause seizures so avoid using in patients with eating disorders, alcohol withdrawal seizures, or seizure disorders
- Trazodone: S agonist and reuptake inhibitor, approved for depression and insomnia; may cause priapism (prolonged and painful erection)
- Mirtazapine: classified as tetracyclic antidepressant, approved for depression and insomnia; weight gain is main side effect

TCAs

- Inhibit reuptake of NE, S, and dopamine
- Include nortriptyline, amitriptyline, imipramine, desipramine, clomipramine, etc.
- Adverse effects: (especially tertiary TCAs) significant sedation, orthostatic hypotension, and anticholinergic effects. They are the most dangerous antidepressants in overdose.

MAOIs

- Inhibit MAO-A and/or MAO-B in the CNS and have antidepressant efficacy
- Differ by the type of inhibition (i.e., reversible or irreversible), the severity of adverse effects, and the specificity of inhibition (MAO-A or -B)
- Include phenelzine, tranylcypromine, and isocarboxazid
- **Selegiline:** selective inhibitor of MAO-B; currently approved only for treatment of Parkinson's disease
- **Indications:** Second-line treatment for major depressive disorder, depressive disorders with atypical features, and some anxiety disorders.
- **Hypertensive crisis:** may occur with tyramine-rich foods or if certain other medications are ingested, including nasal decongestants, antiasthmatic medications, and amphetamines. Avoid red wine, aged cheese, and chocolate.
- **Adverse effects:** sedation, weight gain, orthostatic hypotension, liver toxicity (with hydrazine MAOIs), and sexual dysfunction.

ELECTROCONVULSIVE THERAPY (ECT)

Indications

- Major depressive episodes that have not responded to antidepressant medication or mood stabilizers
- Major depressive episodes with high risk for immediate suicide
- Major depressive episodes in patients with contraindications to using antidepressant medication
- Major depressive episodes in patients who have responded well to ECT in the past

Untoward effects and contraindications

- Transient memory disturbance: increases in severity over the course of ECT and then gradually resolves over several weeks
- Complications of associated anesthesia and induced paralysis
- Transiently increased intracranial pressure. Therefore, the presence of space-occupying intracranial lesions requires extreme caution.

MOOD-STABILIZING MEDICATIONS

Lithium

Indications

- Bipolar and schizoaffective disorders: First-line medication for treatment and prophylaxis of mood episodes
- Adjunctive treatment of major depressive disorder: May augment responsiveness to antidepressant medications in some patients

Untoward Effects

- Dose-related: Tremor, gastrointestinal (GI) distress, headache
- Dermatologic problems: acne; interferes with patient compliance
- Weight gain: may interfere with patient compliance
- Cardiac conduction: electrocardiogram (ECG) changes usually benign
- Hypothyroidism: 5% of patients develop thyroid problems
- Leukocytosis: usually occurs and seems to be benign
- Polyuria: diabetes insipidus is common and may be troublesome to patients
- Teratogenicity: associated with cardiac abnormalities; contraindicated in first trimester, Ebstein's anomaly (tricuspid valve)
- Nephrotoxic

Toxicity Management

- Keep plasma levels <1.5 mEq/L; optimal 1.0 mEq/L
- Dehydration and hyponatremia predispose to lithium toxicity by increasing serum lithium levels.
- Tremor at therapeutic levels may respond to decreased dosage.
- Lithium levels may increase with ACE inhibitors, NSAIDs, loop and thiazide diuretics

Divalproex

- Treatment of choice for rapid-cycling bipolar disorder, or when lithium is ineffective, impractical, or contraindicated.
- Increasingly popular in emergency settings, may give loading dose
- Time course of treatment response is similar to lithium.
- Efficacy for prophylaxis is unclear.
- Untoward effects: sedation, cognitive impairment, tremor, GI distress, hepatotoxicity, weight gain, possible teratogenicity (spina bifida), and alopecia.

Carbamazepine

- Second-line choice for treatment of bipolar disorder when lithium and divalproex are ineffective or contraindicated
- Rare but serious hematologic and hepatic side effects and significant sedation make carbamazepine less useful.
- May cause agranulocytosis

Lamotrigine

- Approved for bipolar depression
- May cause Steven-Johnson syndrome

ANXIOLYTIC MEDICATIONS

Types

- Benzodiazepines: facilitate transmission of GABA
- Buspirone: S receptor partial agonist

Benzodiazepines

Clinical Guidelines

- Avoid abrupt changes in benzodiazepine dosage.
- Use lower dosages for the elderly.
- Do not mix with alcohol or other sedative-hypnotic medications.
- Consider dependency potential.
- May cause confusion, problems with memory, and falls (especially in the elderly)
- Abrupt discontinuation may cause seizures

Buspirone

- Effective in the treatment of generalized anxiety disorder and social phobia
- Lag time of about 1 week before clinical response
- No additive effect with sedative-hypnotics
- No withdrawal syndrome
- No sedation or cognitive impairment
- Headache may occur.

SUICIDE

Presentations

- Recent suicide attempt
- Complaints of suicidal thoughts
- Admission of suicidal thoughts upon questioning
- Demonstration of possible suicidal behavior

Risk Factors for Suicidal Behavior

- History of suicide threats and attempts
- Perceived hopelessness (demoralization)
- Presence of psychiatric illness/drug abuse
- Males
- Elderly
- Social isolation
- Low job satisfaction
- Chronic physical illness

Emergency Assessment

- Detain until the emergency evaluation is completed
- Take all suicide threats seriously
- Question about suicide ideation, intent, and plan
- Get information from third parties
- Don't identify with the patient
- Emergency treatment decisions about suicidal behavior are based on clinical presentation and presence of risk factors

Psychotherapies 19

Table I-19-1. Psychotherapies

Type of Therapy	Goal	Selection Criteria	Duration	Techniques
Psychoanalysis	Resolution of neurosis	Psychologically minded	4–5× per week for years	Free association, defense analysis, interpretation of transference
Insight oriented	Focus on interpersonal goals	Intact reality testing, capacity for insight	1–3× per week for months to years	Defense analysis, interpretation of transference
Supportive	Support reality testing, provide ego support	Healthy patients in time of crises or very ill patients	Days to months to years	Problem solving, suggestion, reinforcement
Behavioral	Modify learned behavior patterns	Those with maladaptive behaviors or psychophysiologic disorders	Time limited	Relaxation techniques, aversive therapy, systematic desensitization, flooding, token economy
Group	Alleviation of symptoms, change relationships, alter family-couple dynamics	Groups target specific disorders, family and couples, personality disorders, etc.	1× per week for weeks to years	Group specific
Cognitive	Change distorted views of self, world, and others	Depressive disorders	1× per week for 15–25 weeks	Assigned readings, homework, behavioral techniques, identification of irrational beliefs and attitudes

Epidemiology & Ethics

Epidemiology 20

KEY DEFINITIONS

Epidemiology. Study of the distribution and determinants of health-related states within a population. It refers to the patterns of disease and the factors that influence those patterns.

Clinical epidemiology. Study and application of population-based data with patient decision-making.

Endemic. The usual, expected rate of disease over time. The disease is maintained without much variation within a region.

Epidemic. Occurrence of disease in *excess* of the expected rate. Epidemiology is the "study of epidemics" (see Figures 1, 2, and 3). Usually presents in a larger geographic span than endemics.

Pandemic. A worldwide epidemic.

Epidemic curve. A visual description of an epidemic curve is disease cases plotted against time. The classic signature of an epidemic is *a "spike" in time.*

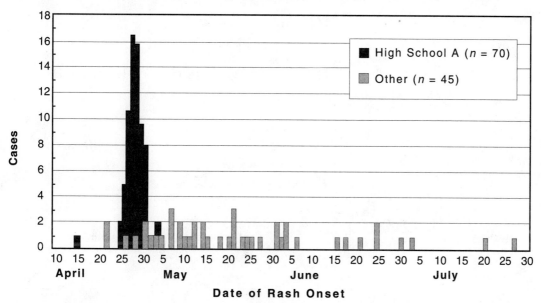

Reported measles cases by date of rash onset, Elgin, Illinois, April 15 to July 28, 1985

Figure II-1-1. Measles Outbreak

An explosive point-source outbreak of measles in an Elgin, Illinois school caused by a single index case whose hacking cough produced an aerosol of measles virus (see Figure 1-1).

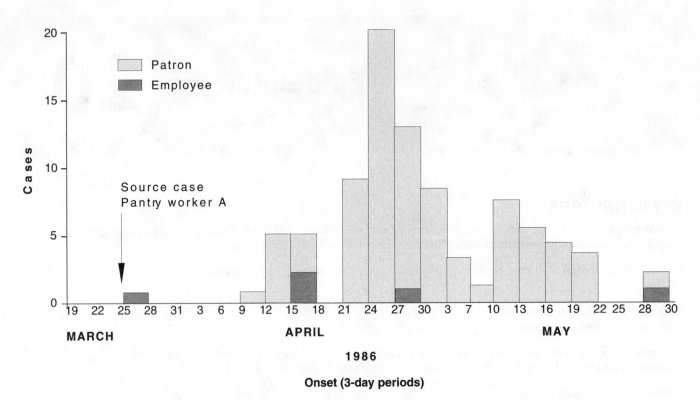

Onsets of illness in patrons and employees: hepatitis A outbreak on a floating restaurant, Florida.

Figure II-1-2. Food-Borne Outbreak

Food-borne outbreak of hepatitis A among patrons of a Fort Lauderdale, FL restaurant (*see* Figure 1-2)

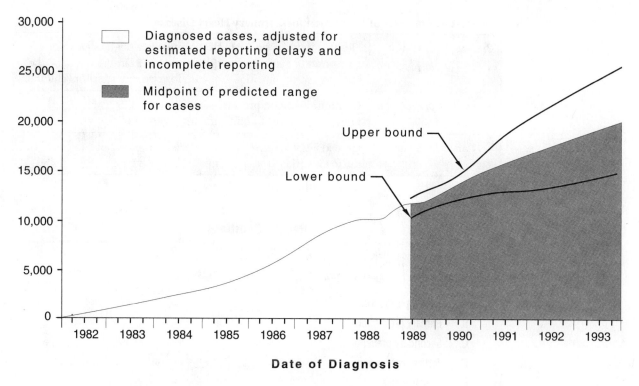

Figure II-1-3. Multiple-Year Increase in AIDS Cases in the United States

Continuous increase in U.S. AIDS cases from the original report of five cases in 1981 through the 500,000th case reported in 1995, and beyond (*see* Figure 1-3).

TYPES OF PREVENTION

Prevention goals in medicine promote health, preserve health, restore health when it is impaired, and minimize suffering and distress. These goals aim to minimize both morbidity and mortality.

Primary prevention is the promotion of health at both individual and community levels by facilitating health-enhancing behaviors, preventing the onset of risk behaviors, and diminishing exposure to environmental hazards. *Primary prevention efforts decrease disease incidence.*

Secondary prevention is the screening for risk factors and early detection of asymptomatic or mild disease, permitting timely and effective intervention and curative treatment. *Secondary prevention efforts decrease disease prevalence.*

Tertiary prevention is the reduction of long-term impairments and disabilities and prevention of repeated episodes of clinical illness. The goals of tertiary prevention are to prevent recurrence and to slow progression.

Table II-1-1. Examples of Prevention for Coronary Heart Disease

Primary prevention	Health education programs to promote healthy lifestyles and prevent onset of heart disease risk factors. An example would be the "Hearty Heart" nutrition program for elementary school children.
Secondary prevention	Community blood pressure screening. Physician support to quit smoking cigarettes.
Tertiary prevention	Graded aerobic physical activity program prescribed to patients during recovery from first myocardial infarction.

Review Questions

Prevention

Response options for Questions 1–4:

    A.   Health promotion

    B.   Primary prevention

    C.   Secondary prevention

    D.   Tertiary prevention

    E.   Palliative care

1. Breast self-examination.

2. Physical therapy/rehabilitation and ergonomic training program for blue-collar workers recovering from severe back strain injury sustained on the job.

3. School-based sexual health education program for middle school students.

4. Confidential PPD testing to detect latent tuberculosis infection conducted at community clinics by county health department personnel.

---

1. **Answer: C.** Self-screening for early detection leading to early diagnosis and effective, life-saving treatment.

2. **Answer: D.** Rehabilitation following an episode of injury with a concurrent focus on preventing subsequent injury.

3. **Answer: B.** Prevention of onset of risky sexual behaviors.

4. **Answer: C.** Screening to detect tuberculosis (TB) infection, to be followed by therapy to prevent progression to active TB.

Review Questions

Key Definitions

Response options for **Questions 5–7**:

   A. Hypoendemic

   B. Endemic

   C. Epidemic

   D. Hyperendemic

   E. Pandemic

   F. Holoendemic

5. A multinational outbreak of influenza

6. The rapid rise in AIDS cases among drug injectors in Bangkok in the late 1980s

7. The long-term, relatively constant rate of occurrence of colorectal cancer in U.S. women

---

5. **Answer: E.** A pandemic is an epidemic that crosses national borders.

6. **Answer: C.** AIDS appeared suddenly, and the epidemic increased exponentially.

7. **Answer: B.** When disease cases are plotted over time, a flat horizontal line depicts an endemic pattern.

MEASURES OF MORBIDITY AND MORTALITY

Rates

Rate is the frequency of occurrence of epidemiologic events in populations. They are used to compare epidemiologic events among populations.

- Rates allow direct comparisons of "events per identical number" of people in 2+ populations.
- Rates permit comparisons of epidemiologic events occurring in a single population assessed at several points in time.

The rate equation is:

$$\text{Rate} = \frac{\text{Numerator}}{\text{Denominator}} \times \text{Multiplier}$$

where the *numerator* is the number of epidemiologic events, the *denominator* is the number of people in the population of interest, and the *multiplier* is selected so that the result of the rate computation generally yields a number in the range from 1 to 100.

Multipliers

For *major vital statistics*, such as *birth rate, death rate,* and *infant mortality rate,* the preferred multiplier is 1,000. The result is expressed as a "*rate per 1,000.*"

For *individual diseases,* the most common multiplier is 100,000. The result is expressed as a "rate per *100,000.*"

Matching Numerator and Denominator

- Essential rule: Match the numerator with the denominator.
- Match on person, place, and time characteristics.

$$\text{Rate} = \frac{\text{Epidemiologic events occuring in a population of persons at a given place at a given time}}{\text{Defined population of persons at a given place at a given time}} \times \text{Multiplier}$$

SPECIFIC AND ADJUSTED RATES

Specific Rates

Specific rates "specify" a subset of the total population that is singled out for special examination or comparison with other subsets of the population. Use the following formula:

$$\text{Specific rate} = \frac{\text{All events in specified subpopulation}}{\text{Specified subpopulation}} \times \text{Multiplier}$$

Common demographic variables used for specific rates:

- Age group
- Gender
- Race/ethnicity
- Highest level of education attained
- Marital status
- Socioeconomic status

(Populations can be stratified on two or more demographic variables at a time.)

Matching numerator and denominator is the most important concept for computing specific rates. Example:

"Event" of interest:	Cancer deaths
Place:	State of Nevada
Time:	Calendar year, 1996
Rate of interest:	Age-specific rate* for ages 45–64
Formula:	$\dfrac{\text{Deaths from cancer among persons ages 45–64 in Nevada during 1996}}{\text{Population of Nevada residents ages 45–64, midyear 1996}} \times 100{,}000$

*Age-specific rate: a rate for a specified age group

Adjusted Rates (or Standardized)

Definition: Rates calculated after using statistical procedures to minimize demographic differences between populations being compared. Comparisons of rates between two groups may be misleading if the composition of the groups differs on important demographic characteristics. Adjustment improves the validity of the comparison.

The following two cases are examples of comparisons between groups where rate adjustment is clearly essential.

> The rate of alcoholism and alcohol abuse is found to be higher among workers in an automobile assembly plant compared with same-age workers at a textile mill in the same city.

Adjustment for gender differences is warranted. *First, the two populations differ on a demographic characteristic:* Automotive workers tend to be men; textile workers tend to be women. *Second, the disease/disorder is related to the same demographic:* Alcohol problems are more prevalent in men. The higher observed rate in automotive workers may be due to the marked differences in gender in the two employee populations.

> The rate of lung cancer is found to be higher among male factory workers ages 50–64, than among male computer programmers ages 50–64, in the same company.

Adjustment for level of education is warranted. *First, the two populations differ on a demographic characteristic:* Factory workers tend to have a low level of education; computer programmers are likely to be college graduates. *Second, the disease/disorder is related to the same demographic:* The major cause of lung cancer is cigarette smoking. People with lower levels of education have higher smoking rates; college graduates have the lowest smoking rates. The differences in lung rates may reflect expected differences in smoking prevalence rates for workers with different levels of education.

Properties of a board-style adjusted rate problem:

- A significant difference in the rate of disease is declared to exist between two groups. The compared rates are unadjusted.
- The two groups differ on a key demographic variable.
- The disease is known to be related to the same demographic variable.
- *Adjustment will tend to make the observed difference between unadjusted rates disappear.*

Table II-1-2. Disease Rates Positively Correlated with Age

		Population A		Population B		Population C	
		Cases	Population	Cases	Population	Cases	Population
Younger	1/1,000	1	1,000	2	2,000	3	3,000
Intermediate	2/1,000	4	2,000	4	2,000	4	2,000
Older	3/1,000	9	3,000	6	2,000	3	1,000
		14	6,000	12	6,000	10	6,000
Crude Rates	Per/1,000	2.3		2.0		1.6	

Review Questions

Adjusted Rates

8. In the United States, the suicide rate for physicians is significantly higher than the corresponding rate for the general population. What is the most appropriate interpretation of this finding?

   A. Higher suicide rates in physicians are likely to be related to job stress, including life-and-death decision making for patients in the care of the physician.

   B. Higher rates of suicide in physicians are likely to be related to constant exposure to human suffering, trauma, and death.

   C. Physicians have higher rates of suicide than the general population; no further interpretation is possible from the information presented.

   D. While the unadjusted rate of suicide is higher for physicians, failure to adjust for differences between physicians and the general population on socioeconomic status precludes meaningful interpretation of this finding.

   E. The finding of statistical significance proves that physicians are at higher risk for suicide than nonphysicians.

---

8. **Answer: D.** When a significant relationship is stated but the comparison groups have some obvious demographic difference, look for the answer that suggests conclusions may be invalid unless rates are "adjusted" or "standardized" to compensate for the demographic disparities.

   In this instance, physicians are generally a higher socioeconomic status (SES) group relative to the general population. Suicide rates are elevated for high-SES people. Once adjusted for SES differences, the finding of higher suicide rates in physicians no longer stands.

   Note: Strongly suspect any response that claims that "proof" has been demonstrated. No single study can achieve proof. Furthermore, no investigator would be so self-aggrandizing as to claim to have conducted the definitive study. Such a response option ("distractor") is almost always wrong.

MEASURES OF MORBIDITY

Incidence and Prevalence

Prevalence Rate: All Cases

Prevalence rate is the proportion of individuals with existing disease at a point in time (point prevalence). It is the proportion of individuals with existing disease during a period of time (period prevalence).

- The focus is on chronic conditions.
- The numerator refers to ALL individuals who have the illness at the time(s) in question.

$$\text{Prevalence rate} = \frac{\text{Persons with existing disease at a given place at a given time}}{\text{Population of persons at risk for disease at a given place at a given time}} \times \text{Multiplier}$$

Incidence Rate: New Cases Only

- The incidence rate is the proportion of individuals developing new disease during a period of time.
- It is the rate of new disease events in a population during a period of time.
- Incidence rates can be calculated only over a period of time, not at a single point.
- The focus is on acute conditions.

$$\text{Incidence rate} = \frac{\begin{array}{c}\text{Persons with disease onset} \\ \text{at a given place at a given time}\end{array}}{\begin{array}{c}\text{Population of persons at risk to catch} \\ \text{disease at a given place at a given time}\end{array}} \times \text{Multiplier}$$

Attack rate is a type of incidence rate that focuses on a known exposure or risk. For example, if 10 of 100 children who attend daycare A, and 40 of 100 children who attend daycare B develop diarrhea, the attack rate would be 10% for attendance at daycare A and 40% for attendance at daycare B.

"Prevalence Pot"

A "prevalence pot" is a common portrayal of the concept of prevalence and its relationship to incidence. At the first moment of observation, the count of cases "in the pot" provides an estimate of point prevalence. Incident cases are observed over time. These new cases are added to the pre-existing cases. As long as clinical illness persists, cases remain in the pot. Cases leave the prevalence pot in one of two ways, through recovery or death. *Changes in prevalence over time can be determined by monitoring trends in incidence, recovery, and death.*

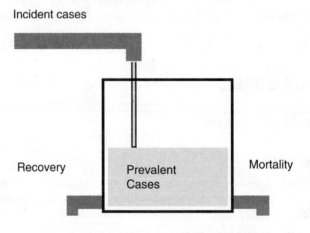

Figure II-1-4. Prevalence Pot Diagram

Number needed to treat (NNT): How many in general population need to be treated to prevent one case?

- The *inverse* of the incidence rate
- If incidence = 16 per 1,000 = 16/1,000
- Inverse = 1,000/16 = 625 = NNT

Table II-1-3. Equations for Common Epidemiological Measures

Measure	Equation	Notes
Incidence rate	$$\dfrac{\text{New cases}}{\text{Total population at risk to catch disease during period of time}}$$	– Acute cases – New cases only
Prevalence rate	$$\dfrac{\text{Total cases}}{\text{Total population at risk during period of time*}}$$	– Chronic cases – Do not include in numerator any deaths or cases that recovered from disease, as they are no longer existing cases of illness
Prevalence	Incidence × duration	– Assuming incidence and duration are stable
Duration	$$\dfrac{\text{Prevalence}}{\text{Incidence}}$$	
Numbers needed to treat	$$\dfrac{1}{\text{Incidence rate}}$$	– Inverse of incidence rate

*Point prevalence will have denominator at a specific point in time, whereas period prevalence will include a specific period of time.

Review Questions

Incidence and Prevalence

9. A pharmaceutical corporation completes trials on a vaccine for a severe strain of influenza virus demonstrating high vaccine efficacy. The Food and Drug Administration approves the vaccine for use in the U.S. As the influenza pandemic approaches U.S. borders, the Centers for Disease Control and Prevention launches a nationwide campaign to vaccinate the population using local public health department personnel throughout the country to ensure that the vaccine is available, free of charge, to all people. Assuming that a high degree of vaccine coverage is achieved, what is the expected impact of this major public health initiative?

    A. Decreased duration of influenza illness leading to decreased prevalence

    B. Decreased incidence of influenza illness leading to decreased prevalence

    C. Decreased incidence offset by increased duration: no change in prevalence

    D. No change in observed incidence or duration: no change in prevalence

    E. Effects on prevalence cannot be determined from the information provided

10. A new, effective treatment for a common disease, leading to complete cure, is developed. Which of the following impacts on disease occurrence is expected?

    A. Decreased duration of illness, leading to decreased prevalence

    B. Decreased incidence of illness, leading to decreased prevalence

    C. Decreased incidence and duration of illness, leading to decreased prevalence

    D. No change in observed incidence or duration: no change in prevalence

    E. Effects on prevalence cannot be determined from the information provided

---

9. **Answer: B.** Vaccination decreases the likelihood of development of new infection and clinical disease. In turn, the prevalence during the peak of the influenza season will be decreased.

10. **Answer: A.** An effective treatment will move people more quickly toward recovery. Average duration of illness will decrease. Prevalence, the proportion of people ill with the disease at a point in time, will also decrease. This will apply to both acute and chronic diseases. When implementing a new treatment, incidence is not affected for a chronic disease. Also, the treatment per se will not affect incidence for an acute disease.

Review Questions

Questions 11–14

Among 245 college students who dedicated one month of summer break to building homes for Habitat for Humanity, 12 developed back strains on the job. Based on the diagram of these 12 episodes of back strain, answer the following questions:

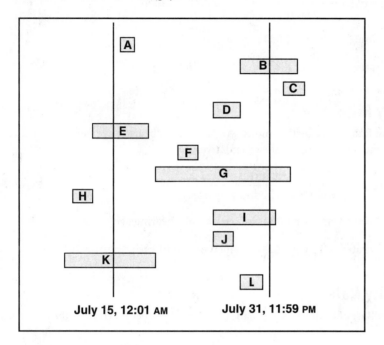

Response options for Questions 11–14:

A. 2/242	E. 3/245	I. 10/244	
B. 2/244	F. 8/242	J. 10/245	
C. 2/245	G. 8/244	K. 12/245	
D. 3/242	H. 8/245		

11. What is the point prevalence rate on July 15, 12:01 AM?

12. What is the point prevalence rate on July 31, 11:59 PM?

13. What is the incidence rate for the period July 15–July 31?

14. What is the period prevalence for July 15–July 31?

11. **Answer: C.** On July 15, two students had symptoms of back strain (E, K).

12. **Answer: E.** On July 31, three students had symptoms of back strain (B, G, I).

13. **Answer: H.** Eight new cases of back strain had onset between July 15 and July 31 (A, B, D, F, G, I, J, L).

14. **Answer: J.** A total of 10 students had symptoms of back strain at some time during the period July 15–July 31, including two with onset prior to July 15 (E, K) and eight with onset during the period July 15–31 (A, B, D, F, G, I, J, L).

VITAL STATISTICS AND RATES

Birth Rate

Definition: Rate of live births in a population during a time period (usually the calendar year).

Simple formula: $\dfrac{\text{Live births}}{\text{Population}} \times 1{,}000$

Interpretation: "Births per 1,000 population"

U.S. birth rate: 13.0 births/1,000 population (in 2010)

Fertility Rate

Definition: Rate of live births among women of childbearing age (ages 15–44) in a population during a time period (usually the calendar year).

Simple formula: $\dfrac{\text{Live births}}{\text{Women of childbearing age}} \times 1{,}000$

Interpretation: "Births per 1,000 women of child-bearing age"

U.S. fertility rate: 64.1 births/1,000 women of child-bearing age (in 2010)

Mortality Rate

Definition: Rate of deaths in a population during a time period (usually the calendar year).

Simple formula: $\dfrac{\text{Deaths}}{\text{Population}} \times 1{,}000$

Interpretation: "Deaths per 1,000 population."

Synonyms: death rate, crude death rate

U.S. mortality rate: 8.4 deaths/1,000 population (in 2010)

Infant Mortality Rate

Definition: Yearly rate of deaths among children age <1 in relation to the number of live births during the same year. Within a population, the infant mortality rate is a key indication of the population's health status.

Simple formula: $\dfrac{\text{Infant deaths}}{\text{Live births}} \times 1{,}000$

Interpretation: "Infant deaths per 1,000 live births"

U.S. infant mortality rate: 6.14 infant deaths/1,000 live births (in 2010)

Neonatal mortality rate: $\dfrac{\text{Infant deaths prior to day 28}}{\text{Live births}} \times 1{,}000$

Postneonatal mortality rate: $\dfrac{\text{Infant deaths from day 28 through day 365}}{\text{Live births}} \times 1{,}000$

Infant mortality rate: neonatal mortality rate + postneonatal mortality rate

Perinatal mortality rate: Stillbirths and deaths in the first week of life/Live births × 1,000

Infant Mortality

Rates per 1,000 live births (2010)

- Whites: 5.33
- African Americans: 12.40
- Hispanics: 5.39
- Overall: 6.39

Top 3 reasons

- Birth defects: 24% of cases
- Low birth weight
  (<1,500 grams)/respiratory distress: 18% of cases
- SIDS: 16% of cases

Other facts

- Blacks have highest rates of infant mortality from low birth weight and infections. Number one killer of black infants is low birth weight.
- Native Americans have highest SIDS rate.
- Hispanic profile is similar to whites, but slightly higher.
- SIDS rates reduced sharply by avoiding having infants sleep on their stomachs.

Sociologic risk factors for children

- Maternal immaturity: Risk of premature birth increases dramatically below age 19
- Poverty is a major risk factor for prematurity and other unfavorable outcomes.
- The single-parent family is also correlated with child abuse, childhood suicide, truancy, and delinquency.

Facts about adolescent pregnancy

- Roughly, one million U.S. teenage girls (10% of total) become pregnant each year.
- Of girls aged 15–19 years, 33% have at least one unwanted pregnancy.
- Fifty percent have the child, 20% have spontaneous abortions, and 30% have an elective abortion.
- *More than half of adolescents do not use contraceptives the first time they have intercourse.*

Consequences for teenage pregnancy

For mother. Often drop out of school. Many never work and become welfare dependent.

For child. Neonatal deaths and prematurity are common. Possible lower level of intellectual functioning. Problems for children of single-parent families can include an increased risk of delinquency.

Adolescent sexual behavior

- Eighty percent of boys and 70% of girls are sexually active by the age of 18.
- More than 20% of all sexually active girls become pregnant at least once before the age of 20 years.
- *Pregnancy is the leading cause of school dropout among girls.*
- Roughly 80% of sexually active adolescents do not use birth control.
- *One out of five teenagers will have a sexually transmitted disease.*

Maternal mortality rate

Definition: Yearly rate of deaths in women from causes associated with childbirth in relation to the number of live births during the same year.

Simple formula: $\dfrac{\text{Maternal deaths}}{\text{Live births}} \times 100{,}000$

Interpretation: "Maternal deaths per 100,000 live births"

U.S. maternal mortality rate: 7.1 maternal deaths/100,000 live births

Case fatality rate (CFR)

Definition: Percentage of cases of an illness or medical condition that result in death within a specified time period.

Simple formula: $\dfrac{\text{Deaths}}{\text{Cases}} \times 100$

Interpretation: Proportion of cases that end in death (fatality)

Example: In a population of 200 people, 25 become ill, and five die from the illness.

$$\text{CFR} = \frac{5 \text{ Deaths}}{25 \text{ Cases}} \times 100 = 20\%$$

Proportionate mortality rate (PMR)

Definition: Percentage of deaths from all causes that are due to a specified cause during a specified time period.

Simple formula: $\dfrac{\text{Deaths from a specified cause}}{\text{Total deaths}} \times 100$

Interpretation: Proportion of deaths from a specific cause.

The PMR is used for the most common causes of death in a population.

Table II-1-4. Types of Measured Rates

Crude mortality rate	Deaths per population
Cause-specific mortality rate	Deaths from a specific cause per population
Case-fatality rate	Deaths from a specific cause per number of persons with the disease
Proportionate mortality rate (PMR)	Deaths from a specific cause per all deaths

Review Questions

Rates

Response options for Questions 15–18:

- A. Birth rate
- B. Fertility rate
- C. Infant mortality rate
- D. Maternal mortality rate
- E. Age-adjusted rate
- F. Case-fatality rate
- G. Sex-adjusted rate
- H. Proportionate mortality rate
- I. Age-specific rate
- J. Sex-specific rate
- K. Age- and sex-specific rate
- L. Age- and sex- and race/ethnicity-specific rate

15. Rate of live births among women of childbearing age.

16. The proportion of cases of a disease that die from that disease.

17. Prevalence rate of obesity in women, ages 45–64.

18. Rate of homicide in black men, ages 15–24.

---

15. **Answer: B.** Restatement of definition of fertility rate.

16. **Answer: F.** Restatement of definition of case-fatality rate.

17. **Answer: K.** Age- and sex-specific rate; prevalence rate restricted to women in the age range 45–64.

18. **Answer: L.** Homicide rate restricted to black men in the age range 15–24.

Review Questions

Questions 19 and 20 are based on the following table:

Incidence and Mortality of Disease

Age	Disease A		Disease B		Total	
Groups	Cases	Deaths	Cases	Deaths	Deaths	Population
0–12	2	1	300	1	40	22,000
13–24	101	34	267	0	30	18,000
25–64	50	42	1,042	2	125	50,000
>64	0	0	986	95	303	30,000
Totals	153	77	2,595	98	498	120,000

19. The case-fatality rate for Disease A is

    A. 77/120,000 × 1,000

    B. 77/120,000 × 100,000

    C. 153/120,000 × 100,000

    D. 153/498 × 100

    E. 77/153 × 100

20. The proportionate mortality rate for Disease B is

    A. 98/120,000 × 100,000

    B. 2,595/120,000 × 100,000

    C. 98/2,595 × 100

    D. 98/498 × 100

    E. Cannot be determined

19. **Answer: E.**
20. **Answer: D.**

YEARS OF POTENTIAL LIFE LOST AND SURVIVAL ANALYSIS

Years of Potential Life Lost (YPLL) (indicator of premature death):

The YPLL for a particular cause of death is the sum, over all persons dying from the cause, of the years that these persons would have lived had they experienced normal life expectancy. Assume life expectancy is 75 years. A person who dies at age 65 would be dying 10 years prematurely (75 − 65 = 10 YPLL). For 100 such people, the YPLL calculation would be: $100 \times (75 - 65) =$ 1,000 YPLL.

- In the United States, the leading cause of YPLL is **unintentional injury** before age 65.

Survival Analysis

Survival analysis is a class of statistical procedures for estimating the proportion of people who survive in relation to the length of survival time. The starting point is 100% survival. In 2000, the median survival time was 78 years.

A survival curve is a curve that starts with 100% of the study population and shows the percentage of the population still surviving at successive times for as long as information is available.

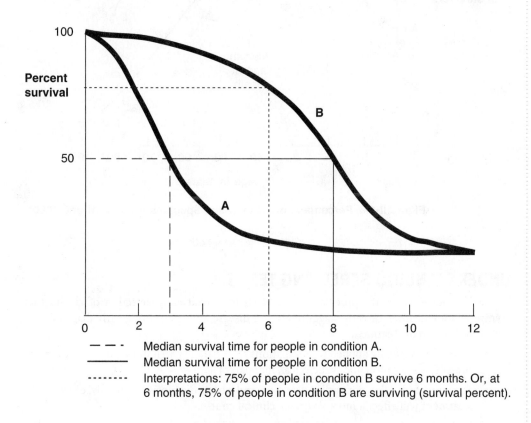

- – – ·   Median survival time for people in condition A.
─────   Median survival time for people in condition B.
··········   Interpretations: 75% of people in condition B survive 6 months. Or, at 6 months, 75% of people in condition B are surviving (survival percent).

Figure II-1-5. Survival Curve

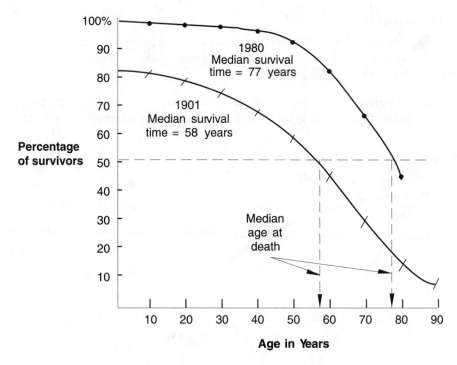

Figure II-1-6. Percentage of Survivors at Specified Ages, 1901 and 1980

UNDERSTANDING SCREENING TESTS

Definition. Screening is the process of using tests to permit early detection of risk factors, asymptomatic infection, or early stages of clinical disease, thus permitting early diagnosis and early intervention or treatment.

- Screening is usually applied to populations of apparently well individuals. Illness, if present, is asymptomatic (subclinical, inapparent).

- Screening tests allow for earlier detection and earlier diagnosis. Hopefully, earlier treatment will effect a more favorable clinical course.

- Screening test results are classified as "positive" (presumed by the test to be diseased) or "negative" (presumed by the test to be well).

Classic 2 × 2 Table

The 2 × 2 table is the standard form for displaying screening test results in relation to disease status. Disease status categories (diseased and well) are diagrammed in the vertical columns. Screening test results (positive, negative) are diagrammed in the horizontal dimension.

Table II-1-5. Classic 2 × 2 Table

	Disease	No Disease	Totals
Positive	True Positive [TP]	False Positive [FP]	TP + FP
Negative	False Negative [FN]	True Negative [TN]	TN + FN
Totals	TP + FN	TN + FP	TP + TN + FP + FN

Cells in the 2 × 2 Table

- Positive (P) and Negative (N) refer to the actual screening test results.
- True (T) and False (F) refer to the agreement of screening test results with the "gold standard."
- True Positives: Diseased people who are correctly classified as positive.
- True Negatives: Well people who are correctly classified as negative.
- False Positives: Well people who are misclassified as positive.
- False Negatives: Diseased people who are misclassified as negative.

Table II-1-6. Screening Results in a 2 × 2 Table

		Disease			
		Present		Absent	Totals
Screening Test Results	Positive	TP 80	FP 40		TP + FP
	Negative	FN 20	TN 60		TN + FN
	Totals	TP + FN		TN + FP	TP + TN + FP + FN

TP = true positives; TN = true negatives; FP = false positives; FN = false negatives

Measures of Screening Test Performance

Sensitivity and Specificity

1. **Sensitivity:** The proportion of people with disease who are correctly classified by the screening test as positive.

   - Sensitivity = TP/All people with disease
   - *Sensitivity = TP/(TP + FN)*
   - Location on 2 × 2 table: left column
   - Highly sensitive tests identify most, if not all, possible cases
   - Important to consider when there is a consequence associated with missing the detection of disease

2. **Specificity:** The proportion of well people who are correctly classified by the screening test as negative.
   - Specificity = TN/All well people
   - *Specificity = TN/(TN + FP)*
   - Location on 2 × 2 table: right column
   - Highly specific tests identify most, if not all, well people (i.e., not diseased), will give few FP results
   - Considered when FP results can harm the patient

3. **Predictive Values:** A measure of the test which represents the percentage of test results that match the diagnosis of the patient. These values are predicted by the disease prevalence in the given population.

3a. **Positive Predictive Value (PPV):** The proportion of people with a positive screening test result who are diseased. (i.e., that a person with a positive test is a true positive)
- Positive Predictive Value = TP/All people with a positive test result
- *Positive Predictive Value = TP/(TP + FP)*
- Location on 2 × 2 table: top row
- ↑ specificity = ↑ PPV

3b. **Negative Predictive Value (NPV):** The proportion of people with a negative screening test result who are well. (i.e., that a person with a negative test is a true negative)
- Negative Predictive Value = TN/All people with a negative test result
- *Negative Predictive Value = TN/(TN + FN)*
- Location on 2 × 2 table: bottom row
- ↑ sensitivity = ↑ NPV

4. **Accuracy:** The proportion of all screened people who are correctly classified by the screening test.
- Accuracy = (TP + TN)/All screened people
- *Accuracy = (TP + TN)/(TP + TN + FP + FN)*
- Location on 2 × 2 table: main diagonal
- Can be used to summarize overall value of a test

5. **Prevalence:** The proportion of screened people who have disease.
- Prevalence can be estimated only if the entire population or a representative sample of the population is screened.
- *Prevalence = (TP + FN)/(TP + TN + FN + FP)*
- ↑ prevalence of a disease usually equals ↑ PPV and ↓ NPV
- ↓ prevalence of a disease usually equals ↓ PPV and ↑ NPV

6. **Likelihood ratio:** The expression of how many more (or less) likely a test result is to be found in nondiseased (or diseased) compared with diseased (or nondiseased).
- Positive likelihood ratio (LR+) is the proportion of diseased people to that of nondiseased people with a positive test result

$$LR+ = \frac{\text{Sensitivity}}{1 - \text{specificity}} \text{ OR } \frac{\text{Sensitivity}}{FP/(TN + FP)}$$

- Negative likelihood ratio (LR-) is the proportion of diseased people to that of nondiseased people with a negative test result

$$LR- = \frac{1 - \text{sensitivity}}{\text{Specificity}} \text{ OR } \frac{FN/(TP + FN)}{\text{Specificity}}$$

Screening Test Diagram

The screening test diagram displays the distributions of the screening test measure separately for people with disease and people with no disease.

The cutoff point or criterion point divides screened people into test-positives and test-negatives.

People with no disease (Figure 1-7; solid line) are either correctly classified as TN or misclassified as FP. Diseased people (Figure 1-7; dashed line) are either correctly classified as TP or misclassified as FN.

The screening test diagram is a useful model of the real world in which values of screening test measures (such as blood pressure) are generally different for diseased (hypertensive) and non-diseased (normotensive) people, but the distributions overlap.

The measures of screening test performance can be displayed on the screening test diagram by identifying the appropriate areas under the curves. For example, the numerator for sensitivity is TP, whereas the denominator is everyone under the curve labeled "disease."

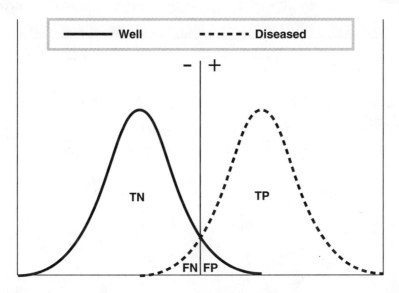

Figure II-1-7. Screening Test Diagram

Table II-1-7. Summarized 2 x 2 Tables

		Disease		Predictive Values	
		Present	Absent	Equation	Notes
Measure	Positive	TP	FP	$PPV = \dfrac{TP}{TP + FP}$	Each value looks at a 'positive'
Measure	Negative	FN	TN	$NPV = \dfrac{TN}{TN + FN}$	Each value looks at a 'negative'
Screening Test Measures	Equation	Sensitivity $= \dfrac{TP}{TP + FN}$		Specificity $= \dfrac{TN}{TN + FP}$	
Screening Test Measures	Notes	Want to identify all possible causes. Use everything in 'diseased' column = TP + FN.		Want to more specifically identify those that do not have disease. Use everything in 'no diseased; column.	

Review Questions

Screening Tests

A new screening test is applied to a representative sample of 1,000 people in the population. Based on the data presented in the following table, calculate the requested screening test measures.

	Diseased	Well	
Positive	90	60	150
Negative	10	840	850
	100	900	1,000

Response options for Questions 21–26:

A.	90/150	G.	840/850
B.	90/100	H.	840/900
C.	90/1,000	I.	930/1,000
D.	90	J.	900/1,000
E.	60	K.	100/1,000
F.	10	L.	Cannot be calculated

21. What is the sensitivity of the screening test?

22. What is the specificity of the screening test?

23. What is the positive predictive value of the screening test?

24. What is the accuracy of the screening test?

25. What is the number of false positive test results?

26. What is the prevalence of disease, assuming screening of a representative sample?

---

21. **Answer: B.** Sensitivity = TP/All diseased people = 90/100

22. **Answer: H.** Specificity = TN/All well people = 840/900

23. **Answer: A.** PPV = TP/All test positives = 90/150

24. **Answer: I.** Accuracy = (TP + TN)/All screened people = 930/1,000

25. **Answer: E.** False positives = Well people who are misclassified by the test = 60

26. **Answer: K.** Prevalence = All diseased people/All screened people = 100/1,000

Review Questions

Questions 27–32

The Centers for Disease Control and Prevention is concerned about optimizing the detection of a disease that poses a serious public health threat. CDC health officials are considering lowering the usual screening test cutoff point from X to Y.

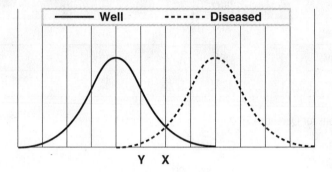

27. Moving cutoff in the manner being considered by the CDC causes the number of false positives to

    A. increase
    B. decrease
    C. remain unchanged
    D. cannot be determined

28. Moving the cutoff in the manner being considered by the CDC causes the positive predictive value to

    A. increase
    B. decrease
    C. remain unchanged
    D. cannot be determined

29. Moving the cutoff in the manner being considered by the CDC causes the accuracy to

    A. increase
    B. decrease
    C. remain unchanged
    D. cannot be determined

30. Moving the cutoff in the manner being considered by the CDC causes the sensitivity to

    A. increase
    B. decrease
    C. remain unchanged
    D. cannot be determined

31. Assuming that everyone who receives a positive test result is referred for medical follow-up, moving the cutoff in the manner being considered by the CDC will cause the numbers of screened people who are referred for follow-up to

    A. increase
    B. decrease
    C. remain unchanged
    D. Cannot be determined

(Continued)

Review Questions (*continued*)

32. At Cutoff Point X, sensitivity is
    A. 100%
    B. 85%
    C. 50%
    D. 25%
    E. 0%

27. **Answer: A.** At Y, FP will increase as more well people are misclassified.

28. **Answer: B.** Although there will be more TP at Cutoff Y, there will be a large increase in numbers of FP. The ratio, TP/(TP + FP), will decrease. A positive test result will be less predictive of actual disease.

29. **Answer: B.** X is the point of overlap and the point of maximal accuracy. Moving to Y will decrease accuracy.

30. **Answer: A.** At Y, more diseased people will receive a (correct) positive test result. They will be TP. TP, the numerator for sensitivity, will increase while the denominator (total people with disease) will be unchanged.

31. **Answer: A.** Larger numbers of people would be screened positive at Cutoff Y and referred for follow-up.

32. **Answer: B.** Notice that Cutoff Point X separates the curve of diseased people into two areas; above the cutoff point, approximately 85% of diseased people receive a (correct) positive test result. They are true positives. Sensitivity = TP /All people with disease.

Review Questions

33. A physician interviews an 18-year-old female patient who mentions that she has just received a negative syphilis test result from the county health department. She describes her sense of relief at receiving the test result. She discloses that she is a sex worker who "works the stroll" four to five nights a week. She has been "tricking" for the past 18 months. Typically, she has oral or vaginal sex with five to eight customers per night. For a higher fee, she will have sex without requiring her customer to wear a condom. On the basis of these findings, the physician is likely to be most concerning with which of the following screening test measures?

    A. Sensitivity
    B. Specificity
    C. Positive predictive value
    D. Negative predictive value
    E. Accuracy

(*Continued*)

Review Questions (*continued*)

34. A 55-year-old man visits his primary care physician with a complaint of urinary infrequency. Examination finds a 1-cm nodule on his prostate gland. The physician orders a prostate-specific antigen (PSA) serum test. By common standards, a PSA level >4 ng/mL is considered abnormal. Using this standard, this test has a sensitivity of 80% and a specificity of 90%. A recently published epidemiologic article found that in a cross-sectional study, 10% of men of this age have prostate cancer. The result on the patient's PSA is 7 ng/mL. What is your best estimate of the likelihood that this man actually has prostate cancer?

    A. 13%

    B. 25%

    C. 36%

    D. 47%

    E. 58%

    F. 69%

    G. 72%

    H. 81%

33. **Answer: D.**

34. **Answer: D.**

STUDY DESIGNS

The following form is used for displaying the relationship of exposure to disease status:

Table II-1-8. 2 × 2 Table Format

	Disease	No Disease	
Exposed	a	b	a + b
Nonexposed	c	d	c + d
	a + c	b + d	a + b + c + d

When epidemiologists observe the relationships between exposures and disease outcomes in free-living populations, they are conducting observational studies. When epidemiologists or clinicians test interventions aimed at minimizing the disease-producing exposures and optimizing health-promoting exposures or factors, they are performing experimental studies.

In **observational studies**, nature is allowed to take its course; no intervention.

In **experimental studies**, there is an intervention and the results of the study assess the effects of the intervention.

Observational Studies

Case report: Brief, objective report of a *clinical characteristic or outcome from a single clinical subject or event*, $n = 1$. For example, a 23-year-old man with treatment-resistant TB. No control group.

Case series report: Objective report of a *clinical characteristic or outcome from a group of clinical subjects*, $n > 1$, i.e., patients at local hospital with treatment-resistant TB. No control group.

Cross-sectional study: The *presence or absence of disease and other variables* are determined in each member of the study population or in a representative sample *at a particular time*. The co-occurrence of a variable and the disease can be examined.

- Disease prevalence rather than incidence is recorded.
- The temporal sequence of cause and effect cannot usually be determined in a cross-sectional study, e.g., who in the community now has treatment-resistant TB.

Case-control study: Identifies *a group of people with the disease and compares them with a suitable comparison group without the disease.* It is almost always retrospective, e.g., comparing cases of treatment-resistant TB with cases of nonresistant TB.

- Cannot assess incidence or prevalence of disease
- Can help determine causal relationships
- Very useful for studying conditions with very low incidence or prevalence

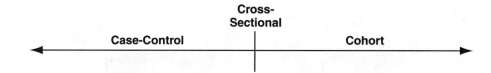

Figure II-1-8. Differentiating Study Types by Time

Cohort study: Population group is identified who has been *exposed to risk factor* is followed over time and *compared with a group not exposed to the risk factor.* Outcome is disease incidence in each group, e.g., following a prison inmate population and marking the development of treatment-resistant TB.

- Allows you to evaluate whether potential risk factors are related to subsequent outcomes
- Prospective; subjects tracked forward in time
- Can determine incidence and causal relationships
- Must follow population long enough for incidence to appear
- Historical examples: Framingham study

Analyzing Observational Studies (measure of effect)

For cross-sectional studies, use Chi-square (χ^2); for cohort studies, use relative risk and/or attributable risk.

Relative risk (RR): Comparative probability asking, "How much more likely is the exposed person going to get the disease compared to the nonexposed?"

- Incidence rate of exposed group *divided by* the incidence rate of the unexposed group. How much greater chance does one group have of contracting the disease compared with the other group?

- For example, if infant mortality rate in whites is 8.9 per 1,000 live births and 18.0 in blacks per 1,000 live births, then the relative risk of blacks versus whites is 18.0 divided by 8.9 = 2.02. Compared with whites, black infants are twice as likely to die in the first year of life.
- For statistical analysis, it yields a *p* value.

Attributable risk (AR) (Also called absolute risk reduction): Comparative probability asking, "How many more cases in one group?"

- Incidence rate of exposed group *minus* the incidence rate of the unexposed group
- Using the same example, attributable risk is equal to 18.0 − 8.9 = 9.1. Of every 1,000 black infants, there were 9.1 more deaths than were observed in 1,000 white infants. In this case, attributable risk gives the excess mortality.
- Note that both relative risk and attributable risk tell us if there are differences but do not tell us why those differences exist.

For case-control studies: Use odds ratio (OR).

Odds ratio (OR): Looks at the increased odds of getting a disease with exposure to a risk factor versus nonexposure to that factor.

- Odds of exposure for cases divided by odds of exposure for controls
- The odds that a person with lung cancer was a smoker versus the odds that a person without lung cancer was a smoker

Table II-1-9. Odds Ratio

	Lung Cancer		No Lung Cancer	
Smokers	659	(A)	984	(B)
Nonsmokers	25	(C)	348	(D)

$$OR = \frac{A/C}{B/D} = \frac{AD}{BC}$$

Use OR = AD/BC as the working formula.

For the above example:

$$OR = \frac{AD}{BC} = \frac{659 \quad 348}{984 \quad 25} = 9.32$$

- The odds of having been a smoker are more than nine times greater for someone with lung cancer compared with someone without lung cancer.
- OR approaching 1 = increased risk of outcome with exposure

Review Questions

Study Design

35. How would you analyze the data from this case-control study?

	No Colorectal Cancer	Colorectal Cancer	TOTALS
Family history of colorectal cancer	120	60	180
No family history of colorectal cancer	200	20	220
TOTALS	320	80	400
ANSWER:	$\dfrac{AD}{BC}$	$\dfrac{(60)(200)}{(120)(20)}$	OR = 5.0

Explanation

35. This means that the odds of having a family history of colorectal cancer are 5 times greater for those who have the desease than for those who do not.

Table II-1-10. Differentiating Observational Studies

Characteristic	Cross-Sectional Studies	Case-Control Studies	Cohort Studies
Time	One time point	Retrospective	Prospective
Incidence	No	No	Yes
Prevalence	Yes	No	No
Causality	No	Yes	Yes
Role of disease	Measure disease	Begin with disease	End with disease
Assesses	Association of risk factor and disease	Many risk factors for single disease	Single risk factor affecting many diseases
Data analysis	Chi-square to assess association	Odds ratio to estimate risk	Relative risk to estimate risk

Table II-1-11. Computational Measures by Type of Observational Study

Measure	Cross-Sectional Study	Case-Control Study	Cohort Study
Prevalence of disease	Yes	No	No
Prevalence of exposure	Yes	No	No
Odds ratio	No	Yes	No
Incidence rate in the exposed	No	No	Yes
Incidence rate in the nonexposed	No	No	Yes
Relative risk	No	No	Yes
Attributable risk	No	No	Yes

Experimental Studies: Clinical Trials

Clinical trials (intervention studies): Research that involves the administration of a test regimen to evaluate its safety and efficacy.

- **Control group:** Subjects who do not receive the intervention under study; used as a source of comparison to be certain that the experiment group is being affected by the intervention and not by other factors. In clinical trials, this is most often a placebo group. Note that control group subjects must be *as similar as possible to intervention group* subjects.

- For Food and Drug Administration (FDA) approval, 3 phases of clinical trials must be passed.

    Phase 1: Testing safety in healthy volunteers

    Phase 2: Testing *protocol and dose levels* in small group of patient volunteers

    Phase 3: Testing *efficacy and occurrence of side effects* in larger group of patient volunteers. Phase 3 is considered the definitive test.

- **Randomized controlled clinical trial (RCT):**

    1. Subjects in study are *randomly allocated* into "intervention" and "control" groups to receive or not receive an experimental preventive or therapeutic procedure or intervention.

    2. Generally regarded as *the most scientifically rigorous* studies available in epidemiology.

    3. **Double-blind RCT** is the type of study *least subject to bias,* but also the *most expensive* to conduct. Double-blind means that neither subjects nor researchers who have contact with them know whether the subjects are in the treatment or comparison group.

- **Community trial:** Experiment in which the unit of allocation to receive a preventive or therapeutic regimen is an *entire community or political subdivision.* Does the treatment work in real world circumstances?

- **Crossover study:** For ethical reasons, no group involved can remain untreated. *All subjects receive intervention* but at different times (e.g., AZT trials). Assume double-blind design. For example, Group A receives AZT for 3 months; Group B is control. For the second 3 months, Group B receives AZT and Group A is control.

Table II-1-12. Comparison of Case-Control and Cohort Studies

Case-Control Study	Cohort Study
Small number of subjects	Large number of subjects
Lower cost	Higher cost
Short time period	Longer time period
One disease: multiple past exposures	One exposure: multiple future diseases
Low prevalence or high prevalence diseases	High incidence diseases only
Major source of bias: recall	Major source of bias: selection

STUDY DESIGNS: BIAS IN RESEARCH

Bias in research

Bias in research is deviation from the truth of inferred results.

Reliability: Ability of a test to *measure something consistently*, either across testing situations (test–retest reliability), within a test (split half reliability), or across judges (inter-rater reliability). Think of the clustering of rifle shots at a target (*precision*).

Validity: Degree to which a test measures that which was intended. Think of a marksman hitting the bulls-eye. Reliability is a necessary, but insufficient, condition for validity (*accuracy*).

Types of bias

Selection bias (sampling bias): The *sample selected is not representative* of the population. Examples:

- Predicting rates of heart disease by gathering subjects from a local health club
- Using only hospital records to estimate population prevalence (Berkson's bias)
- People included in study are different from those who are not (nonrespondent bias)

Measurement bias: Information is gathered in a manner that distorts the information. Examples:

- Measuring patients' satisfaction with their respective physicians by using leading questions, e.g., "You don't like your doctor, do you?"
- Subjects' behavior is altered because they are being studied (Hawthorne effect). This is a factor only when there is no control group in a prospective study.

Experimenter expectancy (Pygmalion effect): *Experimenter's expectations inadvertently communicated to subjects*, who then produce the desired effects. Can be avoided by **double-blind** design, where neither the subject nor the investigators who have contact with them know which group receives the intervention under study and which group is the control.

Lead-time bias: Gives a *false estimate of survival rates.* For example, patients seem to live longer with the disease after it is uncovered by a screening test. Actually, there is no increased survival, but because the disease is discovered sooner, patients who are diagnosed seem to live longer.

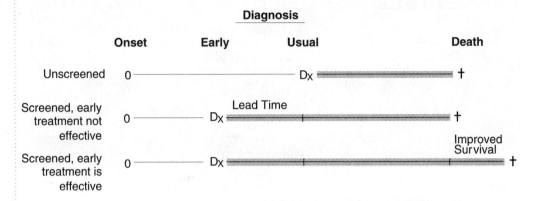

Figure 1-9. Diagnosis, Time, and Survival

Recall bias: Subjects *fail to accurately recall events* in the past. For example, "How many times last year did you kiss your mother?" This is a likely problem in retrospective studies.

Late-look bias: *Individuals with severe disease are less likely to be uncovered in a survey because they die first.* For example, a recent survey found that persons with AIDS reported only mild symptoms.

Confounding bias: *The factor being examined is related to other factors of less interest.* Unanticipated factors obscure a relationship or make it seem like there is one when there is not. More than one explanation can be found for the presented results. An example would be comparing the relationship between exercise and heart disease in two populations when one population is younger and the other is older. Are differences in heart disease due to exercise or to age?

Table II-1-13. Type of Bias in Research and Important Associations

Type of Bias	Definition	Important Associations	Solutions
Selection	Sample not representative	Berkson's bias, nonrespondent bias	Random, independent sample
Measurement	Gathering the information distorts it	Hawthorne effect	Control group/placebo group
Experimenter expectancy	Researcher's beliefs affect outcome	Pygmalion effect	Double-blind design
Lead-time	Early detection confused with increased survival	Benefits of screening	Measure "back-end" survival
Recall	Subjects cannot remember accurately	Retrospective studies	Confirm information with other sources
Late-look	Severely diseased individuals are not uncovered	Early mortality	Stratify by severity
Confounding obscure results	Unanticipated factors	Hidden factors affect results	Multiple studies, good research design

Review Questions

Response options for Questions 36–41:

  A. 520/695

  B. 600/1,000

  C. 520/600

  D. 695/1,000

  E. 80/305

  F. (520/695)/(80/305)

  G. $(520 \times 225)/(175 \times 80)$

  H. (520/695) – (80/305)

  I. Cannot be determined for this type of study

	Disease	Well	
Exposed	520	175	695
Nonexposed	80	225	305
	600	400	1,000

36. Assume the table represents a cohort study: What is the incidence rate in the exposed?

37. Assume the table represents a cross-sectional study: What is the relative risk?

38. Assume the table represents a case-control study: What is the odds ratio?

39. Assume the table represents a cross-sectional study: What is the prevalence of disease?

40. Assume the table represents a disease outbreak investigation: What is the attack rate for people who did not eat the food?

41. Assume the table represents a cohort study: What is the attributable risk?

42. A study compares the effectiveness of a new medication for treatment of latent tuberculosis infection with the standard medication, isoniazid. Subjects with latent TB infection are sorted with equal likelihood of selection to receive the new medication or isoniazid. Neither the subjects themselves nor the clinicians know the treatment condition for each patient. This study is best described as a

  A. double-blind randomized cohort study

  B. randomized controlled trial with crossover design

  C. double-blind randomized clinical trial

  D. double-blind randomized clinical trial with crossover design

  E. double-blind quasi-experimental trial

(Continued)

Review Questions (*continued*)

36. **Answer: A.**

37. **Answer: I.**

38. **Answer: G.**

39. **Answer: B.**

40. **Answer: E.**

41. **Answer: H.**

42. **Answer: C.**

Review Questions

43. A group of 200 hypertensive subjects and a comparable group of 200 normotensive subjects are recruited and enrolled into a longitudinal study to examine the effect of a diagnosis of hypertension on subsequent occurrence of coronary heart disease. Study subjects are followed for 5 years. Final data are presented in the table below. What is the attributable risk for hypertension?

	CHD	No CHD	Total
Hypertension	25	175	200
No hypertension	10	190	200
Total	35	365	400

   A. 0.075

   B. 2.5

   C. 2.7

   D. 0.125

   E. Cannot be computed for this type of study

44. A study is conducted relating percentage of calories from fat in the habitual diet to subsequent incidence of clinical diabetes mellitus. Four groups of inially well persons are selected from the community to represent persons within each of four categories of fat intake. The percentages of daily calories from fat are: <20%, 20–40%, 35–49%, >50%. The groups are followed longitudinally for 5 years and assessed annually for diabetes. The type of study design is best described as a

   A. case-series trial

   B. case-control study

   C. cross-sectional study

   D. cohort study

   E. community trial

(Continued)

Review Questions (*continued*)

45. Alcohol consumption and cigarette smoking both contribute causally to the occurrence of esophageal cancer. These risk factors are not independent; in fact, they operate synergistically. A study of cigarette smoking in relation to esophageal cancer that fails to stratify or otherwise control for level of alcohol consumption would be guilty of which of the following threats to validity?

   A. Ascertainment bias
   B. Confounding
   C. Design bias
   D. Lead time bias
   E. Observer bias
   F. Recall bias
   G. Response bias
   H. Selection bias

---

43. **Answer: A.**

44. **Answer: D.**

45. **Answer: B.**

PROBABILITY BASICS

Combine probabilities for independent events by multiplication.

- Events are independent if the occurrence of one tells you nothing about the occurrence of another.

- If the chance of having blond hair is 0.3 and the chance of having a cold is 0.2, the chance of meeting a blond-haired person with a cold is $0.3 \times 0.2 = 0.06$ (or 6%).

- If events are nonindependent, then multiply the probability of one times the probability of the second, given that the first has occurred. For example, if one has a box with 5 white and 5 black balls in it, the chance of picking two black balls is $(5/10) \times (4/9) = 0.5 \times 0.44 = 0.22$ (or 22%).

Combine probabilities for mutually exclusive events by addition.

- Mutually exclusive means that the occurrence of one event precludes the occurrence of the other (i.e., cannot both happen). If a coin lands heads, it cannot be tails; the two are mutually exclusive. For example, if a coin is flipped, the chance that it will be either heads or tails is $0.5 + 0.5 = 1.0$ (or 100%).

- If two events are not mutually exclusive, the combination of probabilities is accomplished by adding the two together and subtracting out the multiplied probabilities. For example, if the chance of having diabetes is 10%, and the chance of someone being obese is 30%, the chance of meeting someone who is obese or had diabetes is $0.1 + 0.30 - (0.1 \times 0.30) = 0.37$ (or 37%).

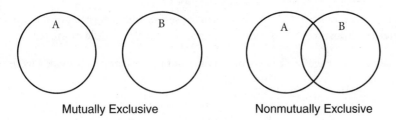

Mutually Exclusive   Nonmutually Exclusive

Figure II-2-1. Venn Diagram Representations of Mutually Exclusive and Nonmutually Exclusive Events

Review Questions

Survival Rates After Surgery

N	1 Year	2 Year	3 Year	4 Year
183	90%	75%	50%	40%

1. What is the life expectancy after surgery? (3 years)

2. If a patient survives for 2 years, what is the chance of surviving for 3 years? (50/75)

3. In an effort to evaluate healthy lifestyle influences at home, a study is conducted to see how many pediatric patients have parents who exercise regularly. Parents at pediatric offices are questioned and it is concluded that 40% of pediatric patients have parents who exercise regularly. Assuming the events are independent, what is the probability that 2 pediatric patients with parents who exercise regularly will come into the office on the same day?

   (A)   0.16
   (B)   0.4
   (C)   0.8
   (D)   0.96
   (E)   0.08
   (F)   0.04

(choice A; this requires the multiplication rule)

DESCRIPTIVE STATISTICS

Measures (Indices) of Central Tendency

Measures of central tendency is a general term for several characteristics of the distribution of a set of values or measurements around a value at or near the middle of the set.

Mean (synonym: "average"): The sum of the values of the observations divided by the numbers of observations.

$$\text{Mean:} \quad \frac{\text{Sum of the observed measurements}}{\text{Number of observations}}$$

Median:

- The simplest division of a set of measurements is into two parts—the upper and lower half.
- The point on the scale that divides the group in this way is the median.
- The measurement below which half the observations fall: the 50th percentile.

Mode: The most frequently occurring value in a set of observations.

Normal Distribution

Normal distribution is continuous frequency distribution of infinite range defined by a specific mathematical function with the following properties:

- A continuous, symmetrical distribution; both tails extend to infinity.
- The arithmetic mean, mode, and median are identical.
- The shape is completely determined by the mean and standard deviation.

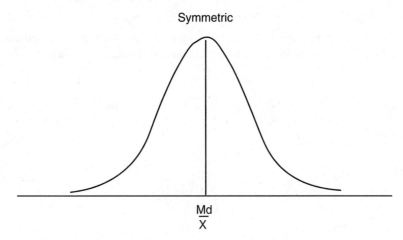

Symmetric

Figure II-2-2. Measures of Central Tendency

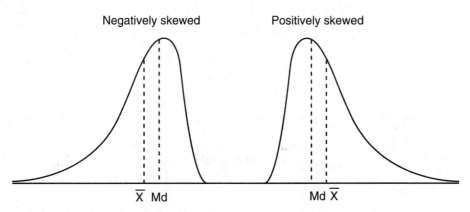

Figure II-2-3. Skewed Distribution Curves

Dispersion of Data

The dispersion of data helps us identify the spread, or the variation, of the data.

Deviation score: The distance from the mean. Found by subtracting the distribution mean from the distribution values you are evaluating. For example, the mean of the distribution is 120 and you want to know the deviation score of the value 150.

$$x = 150 - 120$$
$$= 30$$

This is used to obtain the variance of a distribution.

Range: The difference between the largest and smallest values in a distribution.

Variance: A measure of the variation shown by a set of observations, defined by the sum of the squares of deviations scores of each value divided by the number of degrees of freedom in the set of observations or $n - 1$.

Standard deviation

- The most widely used measure of dispersion of a frequency distribution
- It is equal to the positive square root of the variance.
- Whereas the mean tells where the group of values are centered, the standard deviation is a summary of how widely dispersed the values are around the center.

$$s = \sqrt{\frac{\sum(X - \overline{X})^2}{n - 1}}$$

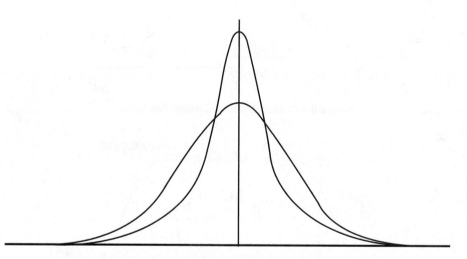

Figure II-2-4. Comparison of Two Normal Curves with the Same Means, but Different Standard Deviations

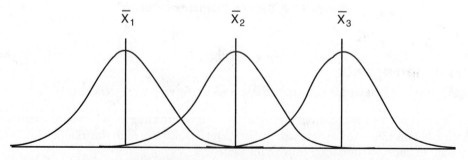

Figure II-2-5. Comparison of Three Normal Curves with the Same Standard Deviations, but Different Means

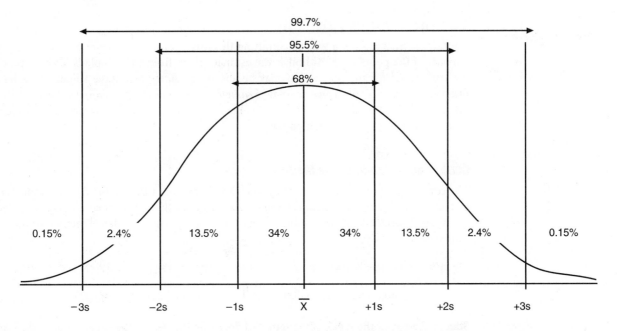

Note: Percentages are rounded so they are easier to memorize. Total area under the curve is 100%.

Figure II-2-6. Percentage of Cases Within One, Two, and Three Standard Deviations of the Mean in a Normal Distribution

The standard deviation (s or sd) is stated in score units. The normal curve has the property that within one standard deviation a certain proportion of the cases is included. The property is as follows: Between the mean and the value of one standard deviation from the mean in either direction there will be 34% of the cases; there will be 68% of the cases between the score at 1s above and 1s below the mean. Within two standard deviations of the mean are 95.5% of the cases. Between 1s and 2s from the mean in either direction, there will be 13.5% of the cases, or 27% for both. Within 3s of the mean are 99.7% of the cases. And between 2s and 3s from the mean there will be almost 2.5% of the cases, 4.7% for the two extremes together. There will be a few cases, of course, 0.3%, beyond 3s from the mean both above and below the mean. You must know these figures. For example: What percentage of the cases are below 2s below the mean? (2.5%)

Students will *not* be asked to calculate a standard deviation or a variance on the exam, but students need to know what they are and how they relate to the normal curve.

INFERENTIAL STATISTICS

Generalizations from a Sample to the Population as a Whole

The purpose of inferential statistics is to designate *how likely it is that a given finding is simply the result of chance*. Inferential statistics would not be necessary if investigators studied all members of a population. However, because we can rarely observe and study entire populations, we try to select samples that are representative of the entire population so that we can *generalize the results from the sample to the population*.

Inferential statistics focuses on drawing conclusions about an entire population (i.e., parameter) based on information in a sample.

Confidence Intervals

Confidence intervals are a way of admitting that any measurement from a sample is only an *estimate* of the population. Although the estimate given from the sample is likely to be close, the true values for the population may be above or below the sample values. A confidence interval *specifies how far above or below a sample-based value the population value lies* within a given range, from a possible high to a possible low. The true mean, therefore, is most likely to be somewhere within the specified range.

Confidence Interval of the Mean

The confidence interval contains two parts: *1*) An estimate of the quality of the sample for the estimate, known as the *standard error of the mean*; and *2*) the degree of confidence provided by the interval specified, known as the standard or Z-score. The confidence interval of the mean can be calculated by:

Mean $\pm$ appropriate Z-score $\times$ standard error of the mean $= \overline{X} \pm Z\,(S/\sqrt{N})$

- Increasing sample size will narrow the confidence interval.

Standard error of the mean is the standard deviation divided by the square root of the sample size. It demonstrates the sample mean deviation from the true population mean.

- If the standard deviation is larger, the chance of error in the estimate is greater.
- If the sample size is larger, the chance of error in the estimate is less.

The Z-score or standard score is a score from a normal distribution with a mean of 0 and a standard deviation of 1. Any distribution can be converted into a Z-score distribution using the formula:

$$Z = (X - \overline{X})/S \ \text{ or } \ Z = \text{Sample mean} - \text{population mean/Standard deviation}$$

- The Z-score distribution is easy to use for calculations because it has simple values. All points in a Z-score distribution are *represented in standard deviation units.*
- Positive scores are above the mean; negative scores are below the mean. Therefore, a Z-score of +2.0 is exactly two standard deviations above the mean; a Z-score of −1.5 is exactly 1.5 standard deviations below the mean.

Z-scores are used in computing confidence intervals to set the level of confidence. Recall that in a normal distribution, 95.5% of the cases are within two standard deviations (2s) of the mean. To get 95% confidence and 99% confidence, all we need to know is what symmetric Z-score to use to contain exactly 95% and 99% of the cases.

- For 95% confidence = 1.96; for calculation purposes, use Z-score of 2.0.
- For 99% confidence = 2.58; for calculation purposes, use Z-score of 2.5.
- Note that a 99% confidence interval will be wider than a 95% interval.

Confidence Intervals for Relative Risk and Odds Ratios

If the given confidence interval contains 1.0, then there is no statistically significant effect of exposure. Example:

Table II-2-1

Relative Risk	95% Confidence Interval	Interpretation
1.57	(1.12–2.25)	Statistically significant (increased risk)
1.65	(0.89–2.34)	Not statistically significant (risk is the same)
0.76	(0.56–0.93)	Statistically significant (decreased risk)

Hypothesis Testing

A hypothesis is a statement that postulates a difference between 2 groups. Statistics are used to evaluate the possibility that this difference occurred by chance.

- **Null hypothesis** says that the *findings are the result of chance or random factors.* If you want to show that a drug works, the null hypothesis will be that the drug does *not* work.
  - One-tailed, i.e., directional or "one-sided," such that one group is either greater than, or less than, the other. For example, Group A is not < Group B, or Group A is not > Group B.
  - Two-tailed, i.e., nondirectional or "two-sided," such that two groups are not the same. For example, Group A = Group B
- **Alternative hypothesis** says what is left after defining the null hypothesis. In this example, the drug actually *does* work.

Significance Testing

To test your hypothesis, you would draw a random sample from a population (e.g., men with hypertension) and make an inference. But before you sample, you set a significance level, alpha, which is the risk of error you are willing to tolerate. Customarily, the level of significance is set at 0.05 and the risk is associated with the rejection of the null hypothesis, even though it is true (e.g., type I error).

Interpretation

p-Value

The p-value and alpha level are very similar, usually set at 0.05, and both symbolize significance. They are only slightly different in that the alpha level represents risk and is independent of data, whereas p-value measures the strength (i.e., significance) of the data against the null hypothesis.

A *p*-value is for interpreting output from a statistical test; focus on the *p*-value. The term refers to two things. In its first sense, the *p*-value is a standard against which we compare our results. In the second sense, the *p*-value is a result of computation.

The computed p-value is compared with the p-value criterion to test statistical significance. If the computed value is less than the criterion, we have achieved statistical significance. In general, the smaller the *p* the better.

The *p*-value criterion is traditionally set at $p \leq 0.05$. (Assume that these are the criteria if no other value is explicitly specified.) Using this standard:

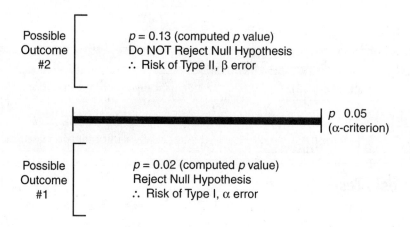

Possible Outcome #2

$p = 0.13$ (computed *p* value)
Do NOT Reject Null Hypothesis
∴ Risk of Type II, β error

p 0.05
(α-criterion)

Possible Outcome #1

$p = 0.02$ (computed *p* value)
Reject Null Hypothesis
∴ Risk of Type I, α error

Figure II-2-7. Making Decisions Using *p*-Values

- If $p \leq 0.05$, reject the null hypothesis (reached statistical significance).
- If $p > 0.05$, do not reject the null hypothesis (has not reached statistical significance).

Therefore:

- If $p = 0.13$, fail to reject the null hypothesis, i.e., decide that the drug does not work.
- If $p = 0.02$, reject the null hypothesis, i.e., decide that the drug works.

Types of errors

Just because we reject the null hypothesis, we are not certain that we are correct. For some reason, the results given by the sample may be inconsistent with the full population. If this is true, any decision we make on the basis of the sample could be in error. There are two possible types of errors that we could make:

Type I error (α error): *rejecting the null hypothesis when it is really true*, i.e., assuming a statistically significant effect on the basis of the sample when there is none in the population or asserting that the drug works when it doesn't. The chance of a Type I error is given by the *p*-value. If p (or) = 0.05, then the chance of a Type I error is 5 in 100, or 1 in 20.

Type II error (β error): *failing to reject the null hypothesis when it is really false*, i.e., declaring no significant effect on the basis of the sample when there really is one in the population or asserting the drug does not work when it really does. The chance of a Type II error cannot be directly estimated from the *p*-value.

β Error can be calculated by subtracting power from 1: $1 - \text{Power} = \beta$.

- Power is the capacity to detect a difference if there is one.
- Increasing sample size (n) increases power.

Meaning of the p-value

- Provides criterion for making decisions about the null hypothesis.
- Quantifies the chances that a decision to reject the null hypothesis will be wrong.
- Tells statistical significance, not clinical significance or likelihood of benefit.
- Generally, *p*-value is considered statistically significant if it is equal to or less than 0.05.

Limits to the p-value

The *p*-value does not tell us *1*) the chance that an individual patient will benefit, *2*) the percentage of patients who will benefit, and *3*) the degree of benefit expected for a given patient.

Types of Scales

To convert the world into numbers, we use 4 types of scales: nominal, ordinal, interval, and ratio scales.

Table II-2-2. Types of Scales in Statistics

Type of Scale	Description	Key Words	Examples
Nominal (Categorical)	Different groups	This or that or that	Gender, comparing among treatment interventions
Ordinal	Groups in sequence	Comparative quality, rank order	Olympic medals, class rank in medical school
Interval	Exact differences among groups	Quantity, mean, and standard deviation	Height, weight, blood pressure, drug dosage
Ratio	Interval + true zero point	Zero means zero	Temperature measured in degrees Kelvin

Nominal or categorical scale

A nominal scale puts people into boxes, without specifying the relationship between the boxes. Sex is a common example of a nominal scale with two groups, male and female. Anytime you can say, "It's either this or that," you are dealing with a nominal scale. Other examples: cities, drug versus control group.

Ordinal scale

Numbers can also be used to express ordinal or rank-order relations. For example, we say Ben is taller than Fred. Now we know more than just the category in which to place someone. We know something about the relationship between the categories (quality). What we do not know is how different the two categories are (quantity). Class rank in medical school and medals at the Olympics are examples of ordinal scales.

Interval scale

An interval scale uses a scale graded in equal increments. In the scale of length, we know that one inch is equal to any other inch. Interval scales allow us to say not only that two things are different, but by how much. If a measurement has a mean and a standard deviation, treat it as an interval scale. It is sometimes called a "numeric scale."

Ratio scale

The best measure is the ratio scale. This scale orders things and contains equal intervals, like the previous two scales, but it also has one additional quality: *a true zero point.* In a ratio scale, zero is a floor—you can't go any lower. Measuring temperature using the Kelvin scale yields a ratio scale measurement.

SELECTING A STATISTICAL TEST

Table II-2-3. Types of Scales and Basic Statistical Tests

Name of Statistical Test	Variables		Comment
	Interval	Nominal	
Pearson Correlation	2	0	Is there a linear relationship?
Chi-square	0	2	Any # of groups
t-test	1	1	2 groups only
One-way ANOVA	1	1	2 or more groups
Matched pairs *t*-test	1	1	2 groups, linked data pairs, before and after
Repeated measures ANOVA	1	1	More than 2 groups, linked data

Meta-Analysis

- A statistical way of *combining the results of many studies* to produce one overall conclusion
- A mathematic literature review

Correlation Analysis (r, Ranges from −1 to +1)

- A *positive value* means that *two variables go together in the same direction*, e.g., MCAT scores have a positive correlation with medical school grades.
- A *negative value* means that the *presence of one variable is associated with the absence of another variable*, e.g., there is a negative correlation between age and quickness of reflexes.
- The further from zero, the stronger the relationship ($r = 0$).
- A zero correlation means that two variables have no linear relation to one another, e.g., height and success in medical school.

Graphing correlations using scatterplots

- A scatterplot will show points that approximate a line.
- Be able to interpret scatter plots of data: positive slope, negative slope, and which of a set of scatterplots indicates a stronger correlation.

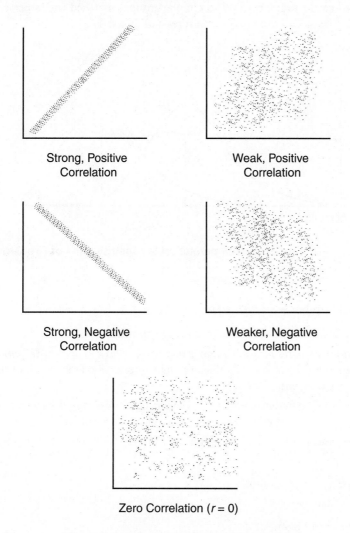

Strong, Positive
Correlation

Weak, Positive
Correlation

Strong, Negative
Correlation

Weaker, Negative
Correlation

Zero Correlation ($r = 0$)

Figure II-2-8. Scatter Plots and Correlations

Types of correlations

There are two types of correlations. **Pearson correlation** compares two interval level variables, and the **Spearman correlation** compares two ordinal level variables.

t-Tests

The output of a *t*-test is a "*t*" statistic.

- *Comparing the means of two groups* from a single nominal variable, using means from an interval variable to see whether the groups are different

- Used for two groups only, i.e., compares two means. For example, do patients with MI who are in psychotherapy have a reduced length of convalescence compared with those who are not in therapy?

- Pooled *t*-test: regular *t*-test, assuming the variances of the two groups are the same

- Matched pairs *t*-test: if each person in one group is matched with a person in the second. Applies to before and after measures and linked data.

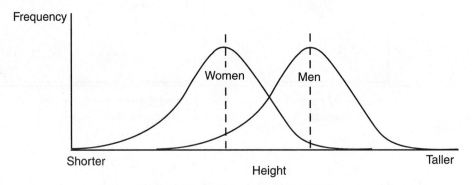

Figure II-2-9. Comparison of the Distributions of Two Groups

Analysis of Variance (ANOVA)

- Output from an ANOVA is one or more "F" statistic.

- **One-way:** *Compares means of many groups* (two or more) *of a single nominal variable* using an interval variable. Significant *p*-value means that at least two of the tested groups are different

- **Two-way:** *Compares means of groups generated by two nominal variables* using an interval variable. Can test effects of several variables at the same time.

- Repeated measures ANOVA: multiple measurements of same people over time.

Chi-Square

- Nominal data only

- Any number of groups

- Tests to see whether two nominal variables are independent, e.g., testing the efficacy of a new drug by comparing the number of recovered patients given the drug with those who are not

Table II-2-4. Chi-Square Analysis for Nominal Data

	New Drug	Placebo	Totals
Recovered	45	35	80
Not Recovered	15	25	40
Totals	60	60	120

Review Questions

1. The American Medical Association commissions a health study of a representative sample of U.S. physicians. Enrolled physicians complete detailed surveys and undergo an extensive battery of medical tests. For a number of analyses, physicians are classified by subspecialty. Although numerous physiologic measures are assessed, the following questions describe analyses of just one of these, mean fasting plasma glucose. Select the appropriate statistical test for a comparison of mean fasting plasma glucose values for representative samples of surgeons and cardiologists.

   A. *t*-test
   B. Matched pairs *t*-test
   C. One-way ANOVA
   D. Two-way ANOVA
   E. Chi-square

2. An experimenter conducts a test of a new medication compared with the current standard medication. Alpha is selected to be 0.05. At the conclusion of the trial, the sample of patients receiving the new medication shows more improvement than the comparison group on the standard medication. The *p*-value is 0.002. What will the experimenter conclude?

   A. Do not reject the null hypothesis.
   B. The new medication has more clinical benefits than the standard medication.
   C. The likelihood that a type I error has actually been committed is less than the maximum risk the experimenter was willing to accept.
   D. The result is not significant.
   E. A type II error has been committed.

3. Body mass index (BMI) is found to correlate to the following physiologic measures. For which measure is the correlation the strongest?

   A. Physical activity ($r = -0.56$)
   B. Percentage of calories from complex carbohydrates ($r = -0.32$)
   C. Systolic blood pressure ($r = +0.43$)
   D. Triglycerides ($r = +0.37$)
   E. LDL cholesterol ($r = +0.49$)

4. A new treatment for elevated cholesterol is piloted on a sample of 100 men, ages 45–59 with total serum cholesterol in the range of 260–299 mg/dL at entry. Following 3 months on the medication, the mean cholesterol for the treatment group was 250 mg/dL with a standard deviation of 20 mg/dL. What is the 95% confidence interval on the mean for this study?

   A. 210–290 mg/dL
   B. 230–270 mg/dL
   C. 246–254 mg/dL
   D. 248–252 mg/dL
   E. 249–251 mg/dL

(Continued)

Review Questions (*continued*)

5. The Wechsler Adult Intelligence Scale–Revised (WAIS-R) is a standardized IQ test with a mean of 100 and a standard deviation of 15. A person with an IQ of 115 is at what percentile of IQ?

    A. 50th

    B. 68th

    C. 84th

    D. 95th

    E. 99th

6. From a published article describing the results of the study presented above, the following data table is abstracted. This table presents the relative risks (RR) of clinical diabetes for each of the categories of fat intake relative to the baseline category of <20%. Interpret the study findings from the tabular data.

	% of Calories from Fat	RR for Diabetes	95% Confidence Interval
Baseline	<20	1	—
Level 2	20–34	1.3	0.8–1.8
Level 3	35–49	2	1.6–2.6
Level 4	>50	3	2.7–3.3

    A. Levels 2, 3, and 4 have significantly elevated risks for diabetes relative to baseline.

    B. Levels 2 and 3 are significantly different from each other.

    C. Levels 3 and 4 are significantly different from baseline and risk elevating.

    D. Levels 3 and 4 are not significantly different from each other.

    E. RR for levels 2, 3, and 4 are numerically different but not significantly different from baseline.

---

1. **Answer: A.**
2. **Answer: C.**
3. **Answer: A.**
4. **Answer: C.**
5. **Answer: C.**
6. **Answer: C.**

SELECTED IMPORTANT COURT CASES

Karen Ann Quinlan: Substituted Judgment Standard

In the Quinlan case, Karen Ann was in a persistent vegetative state, being kept alive only by life support. Karen's father asked to have her life support terminated according to his understanding of what Karen Ann would want. The court found that "if Karen herself were miraculously lucid for an interval . . . and perceptive of her irreversible condition, she could effectively decide upon discontinuance of the life support apparatus, even if it meant the prospect of natural death."

The court therefore allowed termination of life support, not because the father asked, but because it held that the father's request was most likely the expression of Karen Ann's own wishes.

Substituted judgment begins with the premise that decisions belong to the competent patient by virtue of the rights of autonomy and privacy. In this case, however, the patient is unable to decide, and a decision-maker who is the best representative of the patient's wishes must be substituted. In legal terms, the patient has the right to decide but is incompetent to do so. Therefore, the decision is made for the patient on the basis of the best estimate of his or her subjective wishes.

Note the key here is *not* who is the closest next of kin, but who is most likely to represent the patient's own wishes.

Brother Fox *(Eichner vs Dillon)*: Best Interest Standard

The New York Court of Appeals, in its decision of *Eichner vs Dillon,* held that trying to determine what a never-competent patient would have decided is practically impossible. Obviously, it is difficult to ascertain the actual (subjective) wishes of incompetents.

Therefore, if the patient has always been incompetent, or no one knows the patient well enough to render substituted judgment, the use of substituted judgment standard is questionable, at best.

Under these circumstances, decisions are made for the patient using the **best interest standard**. The object of the standard is to decide what a hypothetical "reasonable person" would decide to do after weighing the benefits and burdens of each course of action.

Note here the issue of who makes the decision is less important. All persons applying the best-interest standard should come to the same conclusions.

SELECTED IMPORTANT COURT CASES (*Continued*)

Infant Doe: Foregoing Lifesaving Surgery, Parents Withholding Treatment

As a general rule, parents cannot withhold life- or limb-saving treatment from their children. Yet, in this exceptional case they did.

Baby Boy Doe was born with Down syndrome (trisomy 21) and with a tracheoesophageal fistula. The infant's parents were informed that surgery to correct his fistula would have "an even chance of success." Left untreated, the fistula would soon lead to the infant's death from starvation or pneumonia. The parents, who also had two healthy children, chose to withhold food and treatment and "let nature take its course."

Court action to remove the infant from his parents' custody (and permit the surgery) was sought by the county prosecutor. The court denied such action, and the Indiana Supreme Court declined to review the lower court's ruling. Infant Doe died at 6 days of age, as Indiana authorities were seeking intervention from the U.S. Supreme Court.

Note that this case is simply an application of the best-interest standard. The court agreed with the parents that the burdens of treatment far outweighed any expected benefits.

Roe vs Wade (1973): The Patient Decides

Known to most people as the "abortion legalizing decision," the importance of this case is not limited to its impact on abortion.

Faced with a conflict between the rights of the mother versus the rights of the putative unborn child, the court held that in the first trimester, the mother's rights are certainly paramount, and that states may, if they wish, have the mother's rights remain paramount for the full term of the pregnancy.

Because the mother gets to decide, even in the face of threats to the fetus, by extension, all patients get to decide about their own bodies and the health care they receive. In the United States, the locus for decision-making about health care resides with the patient, not the physician.

Note that courts have held that a pregnant woman has the right to refuse care (e.g., blood transfusions) even if it places her unborn child at risk.

Tarasoff Decision: Duty to Warn and Duty to Protect

A student visiting a counselor at a counseling center in California states that he is going to kill someone. When he leaves, the counselor is concerned enough to call the police but takes no further action. The student subsequently kills the person he threatened. The court found the counselor and the center liable because they did not go far enough to warn and protect the potential victim.

The counselor should have called the police and then should also have tried in every way possible to notify the potential victim of the potential danger.

In similar situations, first try to detain the person making the threat, next call the police, and finally notify and warn the potential victim. All three actions should be taken, or at least attempted.

LEGAL ISSUES RELATED TO MEDICAL PRACTICE

This section lays out a set of rules that constitute the general consensus of legal opinion. Apply these rules to individual situations as they arise.

Rule #1: Competent patients have the right to refuse medical treatment.
- Incompetent patients have the same rights, but must be exercised differently (via a surrogate).
- Patients have an almost absolute right to refuse. Patients have almost absolute control over their own bodies. The sicker the patient, the lesser the chance of recovery, the greater the right to refuse treatment.

Rule #2: If patient is incompetent to make decisions, physician may rely on advance directives.
- Advance directives can be oral.
- Living will: written document expressing wishes
  - Care facilities must provide information at time of admission
  - Responsibility of the institution, not the physician
  - Only applies to end-of-life care
- Health power of attorney: designating the surrogate decision-maker
  - "Speaks with the patient's voice"
  - Beats all other decision rules
- In end-of-life circumstances, if power of attorney person *directly* contradicts the living will, follow the living will.

Rule #3: Assume that the patient is competent unless clear behavioral evidence indicates otherwise.
- Competence is a legal, not a medical issue.
- A diagnosis, by itself, tells you little about a patient's competence.
- Clear behavioral evidence would be:
  - Patient is grossly psychotic and dysfunctional
  - Patient's physical or mental state prevents simple communication
- If you are unsure, assume the patient is competent. The patient does not have to prove to you that he is competent. You have to have clear evidence to assume that he is not.

Rule #4: When surrogates make decisions for a patient, they should use the following criteria and in this order:
- Subjective standard
  - Actual intent, advance directive
  - What did the patient say in the past?
- Substituted judgment
  - Who best represents the patient?
  - What would patient say if he or she could?
- Best-interest standard
  - Burdens versus benefits
  - Interests of patient, not preferences of the decision-maker

Note

Family matters only to the degree that reflects the patient's wishes. Family's own wishes are not relevant.

Rule #5: Feeding tube is a medical treatment and can be withdrawn at the patient's request.
- Not considered killing the patient, but stopping treatment at patient's request.
- A competent person can refuse even lifesaving hydration and nutrition.

Rule #6: Do nothing to actively assist the patient to die sooner.
- Active euthanasia and assisted suicide are on difficult ground.
    - Passive, i.e., allowing to die = OK
    - Active, i.e., killing = NOT OK
- On the other hand, do all you can to reduce the patient's suffering (e.g., giving pain medication).

Rule #7: The physician decides when the patient is dead.
- If the physician thinks continued treatment is futile (the patient has shown no improvement), but the surrogate insists on continued treatment, the treatment should continue.
- If there are no more treatment options (the patient is cortically dead), and the family insists on treatment, there is nothing the physician can do; treatment must stop.

Rule #8: Never abandon a patient.
- Lack of financial resources or lack of results are never reasons to stop treatment of a patient.
- An annoying or difficult patient is still your patient.
- You can not ever threaten abandonment.

Rule #9: Keep the physician–patient relationship within bounds.
- Intimate social contact with anyone who is or has been a patient is prohibited. AMA guidelines say, "for at least 2 years."
- Do not date parents of pediatric patients or children of geriatric patients.
- Do not treat friends or family.
- Do not prescribe for colleagues unless a physician/patient relationship exists.
- If patients are inappropriate, gently but clearly let them know what acceptable behavior would be.
- Any gift from a patient beyond a small token should be declined.

Rule #10 Stop harm from happening
- Beyond "do no harm," you must stop anyone from hurting himself or others.
- Take whatever action is required to prevent harm.
- Harm can be spreading disease, physical assault, psychological abuse, neglect, infliction of pain or anything which produces notable disress.
- You must also protect your patient, or anyone not your patient, from being hurt by another.

Rule #11: Always obtain informed consent.

- Full, informed consent requires that the patient has received and understood five pieces of information:

  - Nature of procedure

  - Purpose or rationale

  - Benefits

  - Risks

  - Availability of alternatives

- Four exceptions to informed consent:

  - Emergency

  - Waiver by patient

  - Patient is incompetent

  - Therapeutic privilege (unconscious, confused, physician deprives patient of autonomy in interest of health)

- Gag clauses that prohibit a physician from discussing treatment options that are not approved violate informed consent and are illegal.

- Consent can be oral.

- A signed paper the patient has not read or does not understand does NOT constitute informed consent.

- Written consent can be revoked orally at any time.

Rule #12: Special rules apply with children.

- Children younger than 18 years are minors and are legally incompetent.

- Exceptions: emancipated minors

  - If older than 13 years and taking care of self, i.e., living alone, treat as an adult.

  - Marriage makes a child emancipated, as does serving in the military.

  - Pregnancy or giving birth, in most cases, does not.

- Partial emancipation

  - Many states have special ages of consent: generally age 14 and older

  - For certain issues only:

    - Substance drug treatment

    - Prenatal care

    - Sexually transmitted disease treatment

    - Birth control

Rule #13: Parents cannot withhold life- or limb-saving treatment from their children.

- If parents refuse permission to treat child:

  - If immediate emergency, go ahead and treat.

  - If not immediate, but still critical (e.g., juvenile diabetes), generally the child is declared a ward of the court and the court grants permission.

  - If not life- or limb-threatening (e.g., child needs minor stitches), listen to the parents

- Note that the child cannot give permission. A child's refusal of treatment is irrelevant.

<u>Rule #14: For the purposes of the USMLE, issues governed by laws that vary widely across states cannot be tested.</u> This includes elective abortions (minor and spousal rights differ by locality) and legal age for drinking alcohol (vary by state).

<u>Rule #15: Good Samaritan Laws limit liability in nonmedical settings.</u>
- Not required to stop to help
- If help offered, shielded from liability provided:
    - Actions are within physician's competence
    - Only accepted procedures are performed.
    - Physician remains at scene after starting therapy until relieved by competent personnel
    - No compensation changes hands

<u>Rule #16: Confidentiality is absolute.</u>
- Physicians cannot tell anyone anything about their patient without the patient's permission.
- Physician must strive to ensure that others *cannot* access patient information.
- Getting a consultation is permitted, as the consultant is bound by confidentiality, too. However, watch the location of the consultation. Be careful not to be overheard (e.g., not elevator or cafeteria).
- If you receive a court subpoena, show up in court but do not divulge information about your patient.
- If patient is a threat to self or other, the physician MUST break confidentiality
    - Duty to warn and duty to protect (Tarasoff case)
    - A specific threat to a specific person
    - Suicide, homicide, and abuse are obvious threats.
    - Infectious disease should generally be treated as a threat, but be careful. Here issue is usually getting the patient to work with you to tell the person who is at risk
    - In the case of an STD, the issue is not really whether to inform a sexual partner, but how they should be told. Best advice: Have patient and partner come to your office.

<u>Rule #17: Patients should be given the chance to state DNR (Do Not Resuscitate) orders, and physicians should follow them.</u>
- DNR refers only to cardiopulmonary resuscitation.
- Continue with ongoing treatments.
- Most physicians are unaware of DNR orders.
- DNR decisions are made by the patient or surrogate.
- Have DNR discussions as part of your first encounter with the patient.
- Do not ask the patient about "do not resuscitate" wishes. Explain details of what is entailed.

<u>Rule #18: Committed mentally ill patients retain their rights.</u>
- Committed mentally ill adults legally are entitled to the following:
    - They must have treatment available.
    - They can refuse treatment.
    - They can command a jury trial to determine "sanity".

- They lose only the civil liberty to come and go.
- They retain their competence for conducting business transactions, marriage, divorce, voting, driving
- The words "sanity" and "competence" are legal, not psychiatric, terms. They refer to prediction of dangerousness, and medicopsychological studies show that health care professionals cannot reliably and validly predict such dangerousness.

Rule #19: Detain patients to protect them or others.
- Emergency detention can be effected by a physician and/or a law enforcement person for 48 hours, pending a hearing.
- A physician can detain; only a judge can commit.
- With children, special rules exist. Children can be committed only if:
    - They are in imminent danger to self and/or others.
    - They are unable to care for their own daily needs.
    - The parents have absolutely no control over the child, and the child is in danger (e.g., fire-setter), but not because the parents are unwilling to discipline a child.

Rule #20: Remove from patient contact health care professionals who pose risk to patients.
- Types of risks
    - Infectious disease (TB)
    - Substance-related disorders
    - Depression (or other psychological issues)
    - Incompetence
- Actions
    - Insist that they take time off
    - Contact their supervisors if necessary
- The patient, not professional solidarity, comes first.

Rule #21: Focus on what is the best ethical conduct, not simply the letter of the law.
The best answers are those that are both legal and ethical.

Practice Questions

- Should physicians answer questions from insurance companies or employers? (Not without a release from the patient)

- Should physicians answer questions from the patient's family without the patient's explicit permission? (No)

- What information can the physician withhold from the patient? (Nothing. If patient may react negatively, figure out how to tell patient to mitigate negative outcome)

- What if the family requests that certain information be kept from the patient? (Tell the patient, but <u>first</u> find out <u>why</u> they don't want the patient told)

- Who owns the medical record? (Health care provider, but patient must be given access or copy upon request)

What should the physician do in each of these situations?

- Patient refuses lifesaving treatment on religious grounds? (Don't treat)

- Wife refuses to consent to emergency lifesaving treatment for unconscious husband citing religious grounds? (Treat, no time to assess substituted judgment)

- Wife produces card stating unconscious husband's wish to not be treated on religious grounds? (Don't treat)

- Mother refuses to consent to emergency lifesaving treatment for her daughter on religious grounds? (Treat)

- What if the child's life is at risk, but the risk is not immediate? (Court takes guardianship)

- From whom do you get permission to treat a girl who is 17 years old? (Her guardian)

From whom does the physician obtain consent in each case?

- A 17-year-old girl's parents are out of the country and the girl is staying with a babysitter? (If a threat to health, the physician can treat under doctrine of *in locum parentis*)

- A 17-year-old girl who has been living on her own and taking care of herself? (The girl herself)

- A 17-year-old girl who is married? (The girl herself)

- A 17-year-old girl who is pregnant? (Her guardian)

- A 16-year-old daughter refuses medication but her mother consents, do you write the prescription? (Yes)

- The 16-year-old daughter consents, but the mother refuses? (No)

- The mother of a minor consents, but the father refuses? (Yes, only one permission needed)

- When should the physician provide informed consent? (Always)

- Must informed consent be written? (No)

- Can written consent be revoked orally? (Yes)

- Can you get informed consent from a schizophrenic man? (Yes, unless there is clear behavioral evidence that he is incompetent)

- Must you get informed consent from a prisoner if the police bring in the prisoner for examination? (Yes)

Interpretation of Medical Literature 23

INTRODUCTION

The purpose of this chapter is to provide you with an approach to reading and understanding research articles and pharmaceutical advertisements. It is based on principles of epidemiology.

An understanding of these concepts is fundamental to the comprehension of medical literature. We have sacrificed depth for the sake of brevity since our goal was to provide a few fundamental tools and avoid complexity.

Research Abstract 1

Wedge resection or lobectomy: comparison of tumor recurrence rates and overall survival in NSCLC patients receiving preoperative chemotherapy

Wedge resection for non-small-cell lung cancer (NSCLC) stage I patients still remains controversial with many physicians. The primary outcomes of tumor recurrence and overall survival (OS) remain unclear when compared with complete lobectomy, which has traditionally been considered a far more effective procedure. However, a recent compilation of case reports and case series reports have validated impressive tumor recurrence and OS rates that were previously only believed to be seen in patients receiving lobectomy. Our primary objective was to compare and analyze the tumor recurrence rates and OS for both wedge resection and lobectomy in patients with stage I NSCLC following preoperative chemotherapy.

Methods

We systematically reviewed individual case reports and case series reports from 152 institutions in the United States for patients who first received preoperative chemotherapy and then underwent either wedge resection (248 patients) or lobectomy (329 patients). A propensity score algorithm was used to reduce the confounding that can occur when examining the effects and variables related to both treatment measures. Following the procedures, tumor recurrence and OS was assessed at 3 and 5 years in all patients.

Results

Preoperative mortality related to chemotherapy complications for patients scheduled to have wedge resection or lobectomy was 0.8% and 1.5%, respectively (P = 0.22). Perioperative mortality in patients undergoing lobectomy was 3.8% versus 0.8% in those receiving wedge resection (P = 0.02). During the predetermined follow-up times at 3 and 5 years, overall tumor recurrence (both locoregional and metastases) were assessed:

  At the 3 year follow-up, overall tumor recurrence was 5.9% for wedge resection and 4.2% for lobectomy (P = 0.41).

  At the 5-year follow-up, overall tumor recurrence was 6.3% for wedge resection and 6.1% for lobectomy (P = 0.29).

When comparing the OS for wedge resection with lobectomy the 3-year OS rates were 82% vs 71%, respectively; (P = .09) and 5-year OS rates were 69% v 68%, respectively; (P = .29). Wedge resection was not found to be an independent predictor of tumor recurrence (hazard ratio, 1.23; 99% CI, 0.96 to 1.15) or OS (hazard ratio, 1.43; 99% CI, 0.92 to 1.23).

Conclusion

Wedge resection and lobectomy are associated with similar overall tumor recurrence and overall survival rates when performed after preoperative chemotherapy. However, postoperative complications and mortality are significantly lower in patients receiving wedge resection compared with lobectomy. Since patients generally maintain superior overall lung function with wedge resection, we recommended that wedge resection be performed in all eligible patients with Stage I NSCLC unless there is a compelling reason to perform a lobectomy.

Practice Questions

1. Information from the abstract most strongly supports which of the following conclusions?

    (A) Both wedge resection and lobectomy have lower mortality and tumor recurrence rates when patients first receive preoperative chemotherapy.

    (B) Perioperative mortality was lower in patients undergoing wedge resection.

    (C) Postoperative complications were lower in patients undergoing wedge resection.

    (D) Pulmonary function tests at 1 year were significantly higher in patients receiving wedge resection.

    (E) The overall survival for wedge resection at 3 years was proven to be higher than that of lobectomy.

The correct answer is choice B. You are asked to determine which answer choice is most strongly supported by the information provided in the abstract. In this type of question, the correct answer is found in the abstract itself and the reader needs only to interpret the information. Of the answer choices, choice B is most supported by the information provided in the drug abstract. The statement, "Perioperative mortality was lower in patients undergoing wedge resection" is supported by the data provided in the Results section. We are told that perioperative mortality in those receiving lobectomy was 3.8% versus 0.8% for those receiving wedge resection (P = 0.02). This data shows that mortality in those receiving a lobectomy was almost 5x higher than seen in those receiving wedge resection. Furthermore, the p value is 0.02, which shows statistical significance.

The stated objective of the researchers was to "compare and analyze the tumor recurrence rates and OS for both wedge resection and lobectomy in patients with stage I NSCLC following preoperative chemotherapy." In other words, researchers assessed tumor recurrence and OS in patients receiving 2 different surgical procedures. Since all patients received preoperative chemotherapy, one cannot draw a conclusion about the impact of preoperative chemotherapy based on the information presented (**choice A**). Remember, there would have to be a subset of patients who did not receive preoperative chemotherapy in order for a comparative analysis to be performed.

Postoperative complications (**choice C**) were not discussed in the abstract.

A clinician could reasonably conclude that pulmonary function tests would be higher at 1 year in patients receiving wedge resection when compared with lobectomy (**choice D**). However, this "reasonable assumption" is not supported, as data regarding lung function at 1 year was not presented in the abstract.

Choice E states "The overall survival for wedge resection at 3 years was proven to be higher than that of lobectomy." In the Results section of the abstract, it says, "When comparing the OS for wedge resection with lobectomy, the 3-year OS rates were 82% vs 71%, respectively; (P = .09)." At first glance it may appear to be a correct statement; however, the p value is 0.09. Therefore, the 2 percentages are not statistically different.

2. Which of the following best describes the type of study performed?

   (A) Case-control study

   (B) Crossover study

   (C) Meta-analysis

   (D) Propensity-matched analysis

   (E) Randomized, controlled clinical trial

The correct answer is choice D. You are asked to determine what type of study/analysis the researchers performed. The researchers reviewed individual case reports and case series reports from a number of institutions. After reviewing and compiling the data, they used an algorithm to reduce confounding variables and subsequently analyze the data. Based on this information, we can conclude that the researchers performed a **propensity-matched analysis**. Propensity score matching (PSM) is used in the statistical analysis of observational data. PSM is a statistical matching technique which attempts to approximate the effect of a treatment by accounting for the covariates that predict receiving a given treatment. This type of statistical analysis is used to reduce bias caused by confounding variables. Propensity scores (obtained from a propensity-matched analysis) are valuable when attempting to draw causal conclusions from observational studies (such as case reports) where the "treatment" or "independent variable" was not originally randomly assigned.

Casecontrol studies (**choice A**) are retrospective observational studies used to identify risk factors that are believed to be associated with a particular disease or condition. Subjects are initially classified as having or not having the disease in question and then their histories are explored to identify the presence or absence of any risk factors. Data are usually analyzed by means of an odds-ratio, and interpreted such that if something occurs in the history of the diseased group, but not in the non-diseased group, then it will be identified as a risk factor.

Cross-over studies (**choice B**) are clinical trials in which 2 comparison groups (for example) both receive the drug being tested and the comparative intervention (often a placebo) at different times. This interventional study will generally begin with one group (group A) receiving the investigational drug while a comparison group (group B) receives a placebo. Then, at some predetermined time, there will be a washout period and then Group A is switched to the placebo, while the Group B is given the investigational drug. This study design allows comparison of those on and off the drug, but also satisfies the ethical requirement that everyone in the study is exposed to whatever benefit the experimental drug may provide.

A meta-analysis (**choice C**) will meticulously examine several interventional clinical studies on a particular disease state (or treatment measure) and then combine the results using an acceptable statistical methodology. The results will be presented as if they were from 1 large study. The classical meta-analysis compares 2 types of treatment measures while multiple treatment meta-analysis (or network meta-analysis) can provide estimates of treatment efficacy of multiple treatment regimens, even when direct comparisons are unavailable. One of the key differences between a meta-analysis and a propensity matched analysis is that a meta-analysis is used with interventional studies, and a propensity-matched analysis is used with observational reports or studies.

A randomized, controlled clinical trial (**choice E**) is a type of interventional study where a researcher will administer a medication or treatment measure to one group of participants and evaluate its effects against a control group who receives another treatment measure or placebo. Subjects in the study are randomly allocated into "intervention" and "control" groups to receive or not receive an experimental preventive or therapeutic procedure or intervention. In the "wedge resection" analysis, researchers compiled the results from several observational studies.

The data evaluated was derived from case reports where patients were NOT originally assigned to receive either a wedge resection or lobectomy.

3. The next step in follow-up of these research results would be to conduct which type of study?

    (A) Case-control study

    (B) Cohort study

    (C) Cross sectional study

    (D) Randomized, controlled clinical trial

    (E) Replication in a different biological model

The correct answer is D. In the current study, researchers reviewed and compiled the data from numerous case reports and case series reports. They then attempted to draw causal conclusions from these observational studies where the treatment was not originally randomly assigned. Using this approach, researchers are able to determine if further investigation is warranted. In this particular analysis, researchers identified a higher than expected overall survival rate and lower than expected tumor recurrence rate associated with a procedure (wedge resection) that is believed to be associated better postoperative lung function as compared to lobectomy. Since the results of their analysis essentially showed no real difference in overall tumor recurrence rates and overall survival rates, the next step would be to further validate these results with an interventional study, such as a prospective, randomized controlled trial (RCT). In an RCT, researchers will likely randomly assign patients to receive either wedge resection or lobectomy following preoperative chemotherapy. Researchers will then be able to determine if there is a statistical difference between the two treatment options.

Case-control studies (**choice A**) are retrospective observational studies used to identify risk factors that are believed to be associated with a particular disease or condition. Subjects are initially classified as having or not having the disease in question and then their histories are explored to identify the presence or absence of any risk factors.

Cohort studies (**choice B**) are observational studies in which subjects are classified as having or not having a risk factor and then followed forward in time so incidence rates for the two groups can be compared. Although cohort studies are a type of prospective study, the next step would be to use an "interventional" prospective study, such as a randomized controlled clinical trial.

Cross sectional studies (**choice C**) are observational studies used to assess the prevalence of a disease in a given population and the factors which co-occur with that disease at a particular time.

Replication in a different model (**choice E**) is a type of study generally used in early animal testing of experimental medications. For example, early animal testing for a new compound may involve a small number of rats. Once data is obtained from a single animal test, there is still a lot of information that needs to be obtained and questions that need answered before this new compound (experimental drug) can be considered for human trials. Therefore, researchers often perform several different types of animal tests using a variety of rat species followed by testing in other animal models.

Research Abstract 2

Mekanib improved overall survival and decreased vemurafenib resistance in BRAF-mutated metastatic melanoma

BRAF mutations have been observed in approximately 50% of all malignant melanomas. The most predominant BRAF mutations found in melanoma are those that introduce an amino acid substitution at valine 600. Approximately 80–90% of these mutations are classified as BRAF V600E. Other predominant BRAF mutations include V600K, V600R and V600D. All of these mutations result in heightened BRAF kinase activity and amplified phosphorylation of downstream targets, which in particular includes MEK. BRAF inhibitor therapy (with vemurafenib or dabrafenib) is associated with well-documented clinical benefit in most patients with BRAF V600E-mutated melanoma (and other subtypes). However, resistance to these drugs and tumor progression generally occurs in patients within the first year. It is believed that BRAF mutations stimulate melanoma cell proliferation and survival predominantly through activation of MEK. The purpose of this study was to determine if the addition of the allosteric MEK1/MEK2 inhibitor mekanib (KAP071714) to vemurafenib delayed expected vemurafenib resistance as well as improved progression free survival (PFS) and overall survival (OS) in comparison with dacarbazine.

Methods

This was a phase 3, multicenter, double-blinded, randomized clinical trial comparing the effectiveness of mekanib (KAP071714) in 447 total participants with previously untreated, metastatic melanoma with the BRAF V600E mutation. Patients were randomly assigned into 2 cohorts. Cohort A (222 participants) received dacarbazine (1000 mg per square meter of body-surface area intravenously every 3 weeks); Cohort B (225 participants) received vemurafenib (960 mg orally twice daily) + mekanib (150 mg orally daily). PFS was the primary end point and OS was a secondary end point.

Results

Median PFS was 11.6 months in the mekanib group and 2.3 months in the dacarbazine group (hazard ratio for disease progression or death in the mekanib group, 0.23; 95% confidence interval [CI], 0.30 to 0.58; P<0.007). At 15 months, the rate of overall survival was 78% in the mekanib group and 42% in the dacarbazine group (hazard ratio for death, 0.43; 95% CI, 0.52 to 0.88; P = 0.02). Elevated hepatic enzymes, rash, diarrhea, and hypertension were the most common toxic effects in the mekanib group. Nausea, vomiting alopecia, facial flushing, myalgia, leukopenia and hepatotoxicity were the most common toxic effects in the dacarbazine group. There were 8 patients in the mekanib group and 15 patients in the dacarbazine group who withdrew from the study due to severe side effects. Secondary skin neoplasms were not observed in either group.

Conclusions

Mekanib, as compared with traditional dacarbazine chemotherapy, improved rates of PFS and OS among patients with the BRAF-mutated metastatic melanoma as well as delayed vemurafenib drug resistance. Mekanib should be considered for use in conjunction with vemurafenib for the treatment of BRAF-mutated metastatic melanoma.

(Funded by SMILE Pharmaceuticals, ClinicalTrials.gov number NCT0123456789101112)

Practice Questions

1. Information from the abstract above most strongly supports which of the following conclusions about mekanib?

   (A) In the treatment of select cases of metastatic melanoma, mekanib alone provides higher rates of PFS and OS than dacarbazine alone.

   (B) Mekanib does not produce severe side effects.

   (C) Mekanib produces fewer side effects than dacarbazine.

   (D) Metastatic melanoma patients with BRAF V600K mutations have improved PFS and OS rates when taking vemurafenib + mekanib versus dacarbazine.

   (E) Most metastatic melanoma patients appropriately prescribed vemurafenib and mekanib are likely to complete their treatment regimen.

The correct answer is choice E. You are being asked to determine which answer choice is most supported by the information provided in the abstract. While several answer choices might "look good," you will be able to eliminate the incorrect answer choices once you examine the meaning of each statement. Of the answer choices, choice E is most supported by the information provided in the drug abstract. The Results section indicates that "Eight patients in the mekanib group and 15 patients in the dacarbazine group withdrew from the study due to severe side effects." Of the 225 patients originally enrolled in the mekanib + vemurafenib arm of the study, 217 persons or 96% of the original study group completed the study. Hence, you can reasonably conclude that most metastatic melanoma patients appropriately prescribed vemurafenib and mekanib are likely to complete their treatment regimen.

The statement, "In the treatment of select cases of metastatic melanoma, mekanib alone provides higher rates of PFS and OS than dacarbazine alone" can be eliminated (**choice A**) since the study was not designed to evaluate mekanib versus dacarbazine. This study evaluated mekanib PLUS vemurafenib versus dacarbazine.

"Mekanib does not produce severe side effects" (**choice B**) is an incorrect statement because the abstract only lists a few of the most common side effects. It does not mention the severe (and less common) side effects. These findings are likely to be found in the body of the published study. Remember, this is an abstract and only provides limited information.

"Mekanib produces fewer side effects than dacarbazine" (**choice C**) is incorrect because the abstract only lists a few of the most common side effects for both drugs. It does not outline the number and frequency of occurrence of side effects. These findings are likely to be found in the complete study.

The statement "Metastatic melanoma patients with BRAF V600K mutations have improved PFS and OS rates when taking vemurafenib + mekanib versus dacarbazine" can be eliminated (**choice D**), because the study was only performed in metastatic melanoma patients with BRAF V600E mutations. Hence, the reader cannot draw conclusions about the effect of vemurafenib plus mekanib in this patient population.

2. In the conclusion section of the abstract, the authors indicate that when mekanib was added to vemurafenib the drug delayed vemurafenib drug resistance. Which of the following is the most likely reason that the reader should question the validity of this claim?

(A) Insufficient follow-up of study participants

(B) Insufficient information on adverse effects and drug-drug interactions

(C) Lack of an appropriate control group

(D) Subject attrition

(E) Use of hazard ratio instead of relative risk

The correct answer is choice C. You are asked to determine the most likely reason why one should question the validity of the claim that mekanib delays vemurafenib-resistance. The correct answer is lack of an appropriate control group. In order for researchers to conclude that mekanib decreases vemurafenib resistance, the control group must be vemurafenib alone and the study group must be vemurafenib PLUS mekanib. In this study, the control group was dacarbazine and study group was vemurafenib plus mekanib; hence, there is not an appropriate control group to answer the question "Does mekanib delay vemurafenib resistance?" In other words, there is no data available to support the claim that the addition of mekanib did in fact decrease vemurafenib resistance. Furthermore, the background states that "resistance to these drugs (vemurafenib and dabrafenib) and tumor progression generally occurs in patients within the first year" and the Results section states that the median PFS was 11.6 months in the mekanib group. The median PFS is a little less than a year; hence, the reader should actually question if mekanib actually provided any benefit at all.

The Results section provides information about median PFS and survival rates at 15 months. The length of the study was sufficient to assess the effects it was designed to assess (**choice A**).

The Results section provides information on adverse effects but does not provide any information on drug-drug interactions (**choice B**). Although a drug interaction could potentially decrease the effectiveness of mekanib, the most likely reason to question the validity of the claim (in the question stem) is because of a lack of an appropriate control group.

The Results section states that "Eight patients in the mekanib group and 15 patients in the dacarbazine group withdrew from the study due to severe side effects." Out of an original 447 patients, only 23 patients withdrew from the study. Hence, the subject attrition rate is low for this study (**choice D**).

By definition, the hazard ratio is a measure of relative risk over time in situations where the researchers are interested not only in the total number of events, but also in the timing of these events. For example, the event of interest may be subject death or it could be a non-fatal event such as readmission or symptom change. The use of a hazard ratio in this particular study is appropriate (**choice E**).

3. In the background section of the abstract, researchers state that purpose of the study was to determine if the addition of the allosteric MEK1/MEK2 inhibitor mekanib (KAP071714) to vemurafenib-delayed drug resistance as well as improved progression free survival (PFS) and overall survival (OS) in comparison to dacarbazine. Which of the following study design changes could have been made to appropriately evaluate all the specified outcomes?

    (A) Add a vemurafenib-only cohort to the study

    (B) Prescribe all 3 medications to each participant but at different dosage ranges

    (C) Replace the dacarbazine cohort with a vemurafenib-only cohort

    (D) Use a crossover study instead of a randomized clinical trial

    (E) No changes were needed since the study was properly designed to meet the specified outcomes

The correct answer is choice C. You are asked to determine what changes could have been made to the original study design so that the 3 initial study outcomes could be appropriately evaluated. Based on the purpose outlined in the question stem, the 3 outcomes being evaluated are as follows:

1. Decreased vemurafenib resistance when mekanib is added
2. Improved PFS for vemurafenib + mekanib compared to dacarbazine
3. Improved OS for vemurafenib + mekanib compared to dacarbazine

The current study design appropriately evaluates PFS and OS between vemurafenib + mekanib AND dacarbazine because participants were administered either vemurafenib + mekanib OR dacarbazine. However, the only way to assess whether mekanib decreases vemurafenib-resistance is to evaluate this regimen against a vemurafenib-only cohort. Hence, in order to appropriately evaluate all 3 outcomes described in the question stem, there would need to be 3 cohorts:

1. Dacarbazine only
2. Vemurafenib only
3. Vemurafenib + mekanib

If researchers prescribed all 3 medications to each participant but at different dosage ranges (**choice B**), then none of the initial 3 outcomes could have been measured because there is no comparison against either dacarbazine only or vemurafenib only.

If researchers replaced the dacarbazine cohort with a vemurafenib-only cohort (**choice C**), then researchers would be able to assess the "resistance outcome." However, they would not be able to assess the effects of mekanib + vemurafenib against dacarbazine.

In cross-over studies, all subjects receive both interventions unless it is a placebo-controlled study then all participants receive treatment and placebo. If a crossover study design were used with the existing study, then group A (for example) would receive dacarbazine only and group B would receive vemurafenib + mekanib. Then at some predetermined point there would be a washout period, and group B would receive dacarbazine only and group A would receive vemurafenib + mekanib. This type of study design (**choice D**) would not be able to assess the "vemurafenib resistance outcome" as outlined above.

Pharmaceutical Ad 1

Tazofect

(tanzopanib 10 and 20 mg capsules)

For newly diagnosed and treatment-resistant EGFR-mutated NSCLC, an effective treatment is now available to improve progression-free survival (PFS)!

- Tazofect is indicated for treatment of EGFR-mutated NSCLC

- Tazofect has shown efficacy in PIK3CA, PTEN, and KRAS-mutated NSCLC

Tazofect is like extra time in a capsule...

...so your patients have more time to do what they want to do!

Tazofect has been proven to:

- Increase PFS by an average of 9 months in all NSCLC study participants (first-line and erlotinib resistant)

- Increase PFS by an average of 10 months in first line NSCLC study participants over those receiving Tarceva® (erlotinib)

- Almost double the PFS in carboplatin resistant NSCLC study participants over those receiving Tarceva® (erlotinib)

The side effect profiles for both Tazofect and erlotinib were similar.

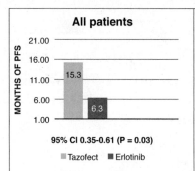

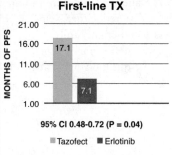

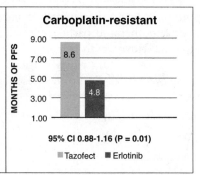

- The effects of Tazofect (10-20 mg qd) and erlotinib (150-200 mg qd) in subjects with EGFR exon 19 deletions or exon 21 (L858R) substitution mutations are presented above. The results were taken from a phase 3, randomized, double blinded multicenter clinical trial. Per protocol, each of these agents was continued until clinically significant disease progression occurred plus an additional 2 months unless mortality occurred. The average follow-up time for patients who completed the study in both Tazofect groups was 17.3 months and 8.3 months in both erlotinib groups.

- Of the 800 initial participants enrolled in the phase 3, randomized, double blinded multicenter trial, 225 (of 398) participants completed the study in the Tazofect group and 388 (of 402) participants completed the study in the erlotinib group.

- Of the original number of study participants, 103 Tazofect patients and 102 erlotinib patients were classified as carboplatin-resistant.

Increased progression-free survival!

Additional product information provided below

SMILE Pharmaceuticals

Smile for life with SMILE Pharmaceuticals

Improved patient outcomes!

HIGHLIGHTS OF PRESCRIBING INFORMATION

Please see Tazofect (tanzopanib) drug package insert for complete prescribing information

Indications and Usage: Tazofect (tanzopanib) is a kinase inhibitor indicated for first-line treatment of NSCLC with EGFR exon 19 deletions and EGFR exon 21 (L858R) substitution mutations in patients age 18 years and older.

Mechanism of Action: Tanzopanib is a kinase inhibitor that acts by inhibiting intracellular tyrosine kinase domain of epidermal growth factor receptor (EGFR) thus resulting in cell cycle arrest and angiogenesis inhibition. Tanzopanib has an elimination half-life of approximately 28 hours in patients with normal hepatic and renal function.

Dosage and Administration: Treatment of NSCLC with EGFR exon 19 deletions and EGFR exon 21 (L858R) substitution mutations in patients aged 18 years and older with normal hepatic and renal function: 10-20 mg daily until clinically significant disease progression.

Contraindications: Hypersensitivity to tanzopanib; use in patients with severe hepatic impairment, active infection and thrombocytopenia.

Warnings and Precautions: May cause reactivation of tuberculosis and hepatitis B. Use caution in patients receiving other chemotherapeutic agents, thyroid disorders, dehydration, mild to moderate renal and hepatic dysfunction

Adverse Reactions:

Common (≥5%): elevated AST & ALT (15%), diarrhea (15%), fatigue (13%), elevated bilirubin (12%), infection (10%), cough (8%), thrombocytopenia (7%)

Less Common (<5%): hepatorenal syndrome (2%), hepatotoxicity (2%), toxic epidermal necrolysis (1%), Stevens-Johnson syndrome (1%), acute renal failure (1%), hypothyroidism (1%), hemolytic anemia (<1%)

Practice Questions

1. The data provided in the drug advertisement most strongly supports which of the following conclusions?

   (A) In the treatment of cancer, Tazofect and erlotinib can be used interchangeably.

   (B) Tazofect is not indicated for treatment of EGFR exon 19 insertion in non-small cell lung cancer.

   (C) Tazofect should be considered for use in patients with PIK3CA mutated NSCLC.

   (D) The combination of Tazofect and erlotinib will improve the PFS to a greater extent than either agent alone.

   (E) The dose of Tazofect should be adjusted in patients with hepatic dysfunction.

The correct answer is B. The key to answering this type of question is to first rapidly scan the drug ad and highlights of prescribing information so that you are able to obtain a general sense of how the content is arranged. Then read the question and quickly search for each of the answer choices in the body of the drug ad itself. In the Indications section of the prescribing information, the following is stated. "Tazofect (tanzopanib) is a kinase inhibitor indicated for first-line treatment of NSCLC with EGFR exon 19 deletions and EGFR exon 21 (L858R) substitution mutations in patients aged 18 years and older." There is no mention of "EGFR exon 19 insertions." That is not to say that the drug cannot be used in NSCLC patients with EGFR exon 19 insertions. However, Tazofect is not indicated (FDA approved) for use in these patients by the FDA. Hence this is a true statement and the correct answer.

Both Tazofect and erlotinib are indicated for EGFR exon 19 deletions or exon 21 (L858R) substitution mutations. Also both drugs are noted to have similar side effect profiles (as indicated in the primary drug ad). However, erlotinib is also indicated for the treatment of pancreatic cancer. Since erlotinib has a broader range of clinical indications and choice A states "in the treatment of cancer," these agents are not interchangeable. It should also be pointed out that almost half of the Tazofect patients dropped out of the trial. Without knowing the reasons why, it would not be advisable to interchange Tazofect with erlotinib. Choice A is a false statement.

Choice C states that "Tazofect should be considered for use in patients with PIK3CA mutated NSCLC." Although the main drug ad states that "Tazofect has shown efficacy in PIK3CA, PTEN and KRAS Mutated NSCLC," there is no data in the prescribing information or drug ad itself to support this claim. Also what exactly does "shown efficacy" mean? The drug may be marginally effective in a small percentage of PIK3CA patients, for example. In other words, there is no data to support this claim in the drug ad. Choice C is an incorrect statement.

Choice D states that "The combination of Tazofect and erlotinib will improve the PFS to a greater extent than either agent alone." There is no information indicating whether the combination of the 2 agents will provide more benefit, less benefit or the same benefit as either agent used alone. Choice D is an incorrect statement.

Choice E refers to making a dosing adjustment in patients with hepatic dysfunction. In the prescribing information section, there is a contraindication for use in severe hepatic impairment as well as a precaution about use in patients with mild-moderate hepatic dysfunction. However, there is no information provided in the drug ad related to a dosing adjustment in patients with hepatic dysfunction. Choice E is an incorrect statement.

2. Consider the following statement: "Tazofect was proven to provide approximately double the PFS in carboplatin resistant NSCLC study participants over those receiving Tarceva® (erlotinib)." When evaluating the drug ad and highlights of prescribing information, which of the following provides the best evidence that this statement is inaccurate?

   (A) Number of patients treated in the carboplatin resistant group for both drugs

   (B) The calculation of months of PFS for the carboplatin resistant graph

   (C) The confidence interval for the carboplatin resistant graph

   (D) The p value for the carboplatin resistant graph

   (E) The y axis data points for the carboplatin resistant graph

The correct answer is C. You are asked to evaluate a statement found on the main drug ad and then indicate what information provided in the drug ad invalidates this statement. Of all the answer choices, the data provided on the confidence interval for the carboplatin resistant graph provides the best evidence that the statement is inaccurate. A confidence interval gives an estimated range of values which is likely to include an unknown parameter (such as actual PFS), the estimated range being calculated from a given set of sample data. In the original statement, the drug company claimed that their drug (Tazofect) was proven to provide approximately double the PFS in carboplatin resistant NSCLC study participants over those receiving Tarceva3® (erlotinib). However, the confidence interval provided with the carboplatin resistant graph contains the number 1. If the 95% confidence interval for a study includes 1.0, then there is >1 in 20 chance that random variation in outcome incidence among the study groups (Tazofect-study and erlotinib-control) is what produced the observed correlation between treatment and outcome. In the instance the p value is also likely to be >0.05. In summary if the confidence interval contains the relative risk of 1.00, the result is not significant. As discussed, this should also lead the reader to believe that the P-value (provided on the same graph, choice D) is also inaccurate. However, without the data seen with the confidence interval, the reader would have no way of suspecting that the provided P-value is also likely inaccurate. Therefore, choice C is the best answer

In the key under the 3 graphs, it is stated that 103 Tazofect patients and 102 erlotinib patients were classified as carboplatin resistant. This is a sufficient number of patients in each group (**choice A**).

The statement makes reference to the number of months of PFS in the Tazofect group being "almost double" the erlotinib group in carboplatin resistant patients. The PFS for Tazofect is 8.6 months and the PFS for erlotinib is 4.8 months. This statement could have been phrased differently, but is not completely inaccurate (**choice B**).

When comparing the data points on the y-axes of the 3 graphs, the y-axis on the carboplatin resistant group was clearly manipulated so that a more "profound graphical representation" of the actual results is evident. Although this should cause the reader to question the integrity of the authors, choice C is still the best answer.

3. Shortly after Tazofect is released for use in the general population, the FDA and drug manufacturer begin to receive numerous reports of complete treatment failure in both carboplatin resistant patients and first line therapy patients as well as higher than expected percentages of adverse events in all patients. Which of the following is the most likely reason for these reports on Tazofect?

    (A) Insufficient follow-up of study participants

    (B) Insufficient information on adverse effects

    (C) Insufficient information on drug indications

    (D) Subject attrition

    (E) Type II error was committed

The correct answer is choice D. In the question stem we are told that shortly after the drug is used in the general population there are reports of treatment failure in both carboplatin resistant patients and first line treatment patients. We are also told that higher-than-expected percentages of adverse events are occurring. The question is asking for the most likely cause of this occurrence. The most likely reason based on the data provided in the drug ad and highlights of prescribing information is subject attrition. Under the 3 graphs it is stated that "Of the 800 initial participants enrolled in the phase 3, randomized, double blinded multicenter trial, 225 (of 398) participants completed the study in the Tazofect group and 388 (of 402) participants completed the study in the erlotinib group." Approximately half (225/398 participants) of the original Tazofect study participants never completed the trial. Furthermore, the authors did not provide an explanation as to why they did not complete the study. Is it likely that they did not complete the trial because of severe adverse effects and/or death?

Without knowing the reasons why the participants never completed the trial, it is difficult to evaluate the safety and efficacy of Tazofect in both first line therapy and carboplatin resistant patients. Also, it is quite possible that only a small percentage of the 103 participants in the carboplatin resistant arm of the study never completed the study. Without more information, it is hard for the reader to make a valid conclusion. In summary, the authors should have indicated why almost half of the study participants never completed the study; hence, the primary reason why these reports are occurring (due to treatment failures and increased adverse effect occurrence) is directly related to the circumstances surrounding the high level of subject attrition in this trial.

The phase 3 trial for Tazofect lasted in each patient until clinically significant disease progression occurred plus an additional 2 months unless mortality occurred. Furthermore, the average follow-up time for patients who completed the study was listed. The length of the study was sufficient to assess the effects it was designed to assess. Choice A is an incorrect response.

At the bottom of the highlights of prescribing information page of the drug ad, there is an extensive list of adverse effects and percentage of occurrence of each of these side effects. Hence, sufficient information on these adverse effects was provided. Choice B is an incorrect response. However, this information was based on the number of patients who completed the clinical trial. Since almost half of the study participants (in the Tazofect arm) never completed the trial, an accurate accounting of side effect appearance was not available. This is directly related to subject attrition.

At the top of the highlights of prescribing information page of the drug ad, it clearly states that "Tazofect (tanzopanib) is a kinase inhibitor indicated for first-line treatment of NSCLC with EGFR exon 19 deletions and EGFR exon 21 (L858R) substitution mutations in patients aged 18 years and older." The drug is NOT indicated for use in carboplatin resistant patients. Although there is a graph on the first page of the drug ad and comments about proven effects, the drug ad never claimed that the drug was "indicated" for use in carboplatin patients. Choice C is an incorrect response.

A type II or beta error is where the researcher fails to reject the null hypothesis when it is really false. In other words, the researcher declared that there was no significant effect on the basis of the sample when there really is one in the population. The likely impact of this type of error is that the drug (Tazofect) would NOT obtain FDA approval and the general population would not receive this medication. Choice E is an incorrect response.

Pharmaceutical Ad 2

GluSense™ ... because it makes sense!

(Glugliflozin 75 mg, 150 mg and 300 mg tablets)

Diabetes is a complex disease ...

GluSense is a simple treatment measure with proven therapeutic outcomes!

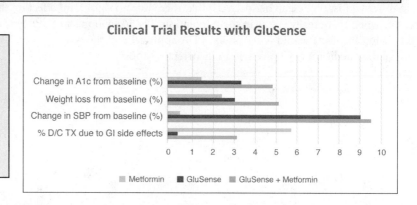

Clinical Trial Results with GluSense

Change in A1c from baseline (%)
Weight loss from baseline (%)
Change in SBP from baseline (%)
% D/C TX due to GI side effects

0 1 2 3 4 5 6 7 8 9 10

■ Metformin ■ GluSense ■ GluSense + Metformin

- The clinical effects of GluSense (150-mg qd), metformin (1000 mg bid) and combination therapy (GluSense 150 mg qd + metformin 1000 mg bid) in patients with newly diagnosed type 2 diabetes who failed to meet glycemic goals with diet and exercise alone are presented above. The results were taken from a phase 3, randomized, double-blinded multicenter clinical trial.

- Each therapy was administered in conjunction with a structured diet and exercise program.

- A baseline A1c, body weight and systolic blood pressure reading were obtained at the onset of the trial and every 8 weeks during the trial. All participants were enrolled in the study for 12 months.

- Of the 1600 initial participants enrolled in the trial, 462 (of 510) participants in the metformin-only group completed the study, 358 (of 533) of the GluSense-only group completed the study, and 313 (of 577) in the GluSense + metformin group completed the study.

- The primary reason (as stated by the patient) for withdrawing from the study was unwanted side effects.

GluSense demonstrated <u>greater reductions</u> in A1c, weight loss & blood pressure than metformin alone at 52 weeks!

- GluSense is indicated for treatment of T2DM as monotherapy & in combination with metformin.

- GluSense has shown efficacy when used in conjunction with other oral hypoglycemic agents.

The treatment your T2DM patients have always needed is finally here!!

SMILE Pharmaceuticals

Smile for life with SMILE Pharmaceuticals

GluSense has been proven to:

- Reduce A1c in T2DM patients by an average of 3.4% as monotherapy (P<0.001) & in combination with metformin an average of 4.9% (P<0.002) – mean baseline A1c = 8.05%

- Reduce baseline weight in T2DM patients by an average of 3.1% as monotherapy (P<0.02) & in combination with metformin an average of 5.2% (P<0.03) – mean baseline weight = 182 lbs (87.3 kg)

- Reduce baseline systolic blood pressure in T2DM patients by an average of 9.1% as monotherapy (P<0.006) & in combination with metformin an average of 9.6% (P<0.001) – mean baseline SBP = 177 mm Hg.

Additional product information provided below

HIGHLIGHTS OF PRESCRIBING INFORMATION

Please see GluSense (glugliflozin) drug package insert for complete prescribing information.

Indications and Usage: GluSense (glugliflozin) is an SGLT2 inhibitor with insulin-sensitizing properties, indicated for the treatment of type 2 diabetes in conjunction with diet and exercise as monotherapy, and in combination with metformin in patients aged 18 years and older.

Mechanism of Action: Glugliflozin is an SGLT2 inhibitor with insulin-sensitizing properties. This agent has a dual mechanism of action. It acts by:

Inhibiting the sodium-glucose cotransporter 2 (SGLT2), thereby reducing glucose reabsorption and increasing urinary glucose excretion

Decreasing insulin in the periphery and liver, resulting in increased insulin-dependent glucose disposal and decreased hepatic glucose output. Glugliflozin is an agonist for peroxisome proliferator-activated receptor-gamma (PPARγ). Activation of PPARγ nuclear receptors in the liver, skeletal muscle, and adipose tissue modulates the transcription of a number of insulin responsive genes involved in the control of glucose and lipid metabolism.

Other: antagonizes peripheral alpha-1 adrenergic receptors

Pharmacokinetics

Glugliflozin has an elimination half-life of approximately 16 hours in patients with normal hepatic and renal function.

Following oral administration of glugliflozin, Tmax occurs within 3 hours.

Glugliflozin is extensively metabolized by hydroxylation and oxidation; the metabolites also partly convert to glucuronide or sulfate conjugates.

Following oral administration of glugliflozin, approximately 15–20% of the drug dose is recovered in the urine.

Dosage and Administration: Treatment of type 2 diabetes in patients aged 18 years or older who have failed to meet glycemic goals with diet and exercise alone:

Monotherapy: 150-300 mg PO qd; start at 75 mg PO qd and increase by 75 mg qwk; max dose 450 mg/day

Combination with metformin: same as monotherapy and standard metformin dose of 2000 mg daily (in divided doses)

Contraindications: Type 1 diabetes mellitus, hypersensitivity to glugliflozin and/or sulfonamides; NYHA class III or IV heart failure, severe hepatic impairment, hyperkalemia, use with medications causing hyperkalemia and diabetic ketoacidosis

Warnings and Precautions: May cause hypoglycemia, hypotension, and AST/ALT elevation. Caution use in elderly patients with poorly controlled diabetes and patients with past history of cardiovascular disease.

Adverse Reactions (for a complete list, see drug package insert)

Common (≥5%):	Less Common (<5%):
Hyperkalemia	Fatigue
Hypoglycemia	Hepatic dysfunction
Orthostatic hypotension	Thirst
Dizziness	Fainting
Tachycardia	Mental impairment
Hyperhidrosis	Pancreatitis

Drug Interactions (see drug package insert)

Practice Questions

1. The data provided in the drug advertisement most strongly supports which of the following conclusions?

    (A) GluSense is a substitute for diet and exercise in type 2 diabetes due to its weight loss properties.

    (B) GluSense is recommended for use in patients with a history of myocardial infarction.

    (C) GluSense is safer to use in patients with type 2 diabetes than metformin.

    (D) The antihypertensive effects of GluSense are comparable to some currently available antihypertensive medications.

    (E) The combination use of GluSense and a sulfonylurea is recommended for those who initially fail sulfonylurea monotherapy.

The correct answer is D. This type of question generally requires a process of elimination. The statement "The antihypertensive effects of GluSense are comparable to some currently available antihypertensive medications" is most strongly supported by the drug ad. Relevant information to support this statement can be found in several places: First in the table, GluSense is associated with 9.1% decrease in average systolic blood pressure. This percentage decrease is comparable to the diuretics, low-moderate doses of ACE inhibitors, alpha antagonists as well as varying doses of other drugs from different drug classes. Second, the mechanism of action section of the highlights of prescribing information states that this drug antagonizes peripheral alpha-1 adrenergic receptors. This is the same mechanism of action as drugs like terazosin and doxazosin. Finally, the side effects of the drug (orthostatic hypotension, dizziness, and tachycardia) also support its antihypertensive properties since these are side effects commonly seen in alpha antagonists. Hence, out of all of the answer choices, this statement is most strongly supported by the drug ad.

There are several places which indicate GluSense is used in conjunction with diet and exercise, such as the key under the chart on the main ad page and in the Indications and Usage section in the highlights of prescribing information. Although the drug promotes weight loss, GluSence is not a substitute for diet and exercise (**choice A**).

The Warnings and Precautions section states that GluSense should be used cautiously in patients with past history of cardiovascular disease. Furthermore, in Contraindications, it is stated that GluSense is contraindicated for use in patients with NYHA Class III or IV heart failure. Since myocardial infarction (**choice B**) is a form of cardiovascular disease and a common precipitating cause of heart failure, GluSense would not be recommended for use in these cases. GluSense may potentially be used "cautiously" in patients with a mild form of cardiovascular disease but is not "recommended."

The drug ad does not have a safety profile comparison between GluSense and metformin (**choice C**). The only related comparison between the drugs is the appearance of severe GI side effects leading to withdrawal from the study.

The only statement relating to the use of GluSense and another drug is found in the main area of the drug ad: "GluSense has shown efficacy when used in conjunction with other oral hypoglycemic agents." It does not specify the names or drug classes of the other agents (**choice E**). Furthermore, it does not provide any data to support this claim.

2. Of the initial trial participants, 175 persons from the GluSense-only group and an even large number from the GluSense and metformin group withdrew from the study. Which of the following is the most likely reason for participant withdrawal?

    (A) Appearance of drug interactions

    (B) Hypersensitivity to sulfonamides

    (C) Severe hypoglycemia

    (D) Severe hypotension

    (E) Severe GI side effects

The correct answer is C. You are asked to determine the most likely reason why participants withdrew from the study. In the key under the graph on page 1, it states "The primary reason (as stated by the patient) for withdrawing from the study was unwanted side effects." However, it is not stated what side effect caused them to withdraw. Therefore, you must determine the most likely reason based on information provided in the drug ad. The Adverse Reactions section of the highlights of prescribing information provides only a "partial" list of side effects with a percent occurrence above and below 5% so this section alone cannot be used to answer the question. The correct answer can be derived from the section on the bottom right of the main drug ad. It states that GluSense has been proven to reduce A1c in type 2 diabetes (T2DM) patients by an average of 3.4% as monotherapy (P<0.001) and in combination with metformin an average of 4.9% (P<0.002). The mean baseline A1c was 8.05% for study participants. If the mean baseline A1c was 8.05%, that means that some patients likely started with an A1c around 7%. Remember that an A1c 6% is an average daily glucose level of 126 mg/dL. If you lower this A1c by 3.4% (GluSense only) or 4.9% (Glusense + metformin), the resulting A1c levels are 3.6% and 2.1%, respectively. Since the A1c is a long-term average of the daily blood glucose levels, it is likely that this agent caused severe hypoglycemia in participants; hence, the likely reason for withdrawal from the study. Furthermore, it is stated that hypoglycemia is one of the most common adverse effects. Choice C is the best answer choice.

The drug ad does not specifically mention any problems with drug-drug interactions (**choice A**) in the clinical trial and there is a comment indicating that the reader should please see GluSense (glugliflozin) drug package insert for complete prescribing information. Based on this information, it is unlikely that drug-drug interactions are the primary reason for patient withdrawal.

The Contraindications section states that GluSense is contraindicated for use in patients with sulfonamide hypersensitivity (**choice B**). However, there is nothing which would lead the reader to believe this is the primary reason for withdrawal from the study.

The bottom right of the ad states that GluSense has been proven to reduce baseline SBP (systolic blood pressure) in T2DM patients by an average of 9.1% as monotherapy (P<0.006) and in combination with metformin an average of 9.6% (P<0.001). The mean participant baseline SBP was 177 mm Hg. Even if the starting blood pressure was 100 mm Hg, the patient would still not be hypotensive with a 9.6% drop in blood pressure. Note, too that orthostatic hypotension is listed as a common side effect, but with the information presented it is unlikely that was the primary reason for patient withdrawal (**choice D**).

It is unlikely that severe GI side effects (**choice E**) were the primary reason for participant withdrawal since the table shows that the GluSense-alone arm had almost no withdrawals from study. GluSense also improved the GI side effect withdrawal rate for patients receiving metformin when the 2 medications were combined.

3. A 64-year-old man comes to the physician with complaints of increasing polyuria and polydipsia. His past medical history is significant for type 2 diabetes, hypertension, hyperlipidemia, and a myocardial infarction 4 years ago. Allergy history includes an anaphylactic reaction to levofloxacin. He is currently receiving metformin 1000 mg 2x daily, enalapril 10 mg daily, pravastatin 20 mg daily, and spironolactone 25 mg twice daily. Physical examination shows blood pressure of 126/82 mm Hg, heart rate 62/min, height 172.7 cm (5 feet, 8 inches), weight 88.6 kg (195 lbs), and BMI 29.6.

Laboratory studies show:

- Blood glucose: 215 mg/dL
- A1c: 10.5%
- Albumin: 3.8 g/dL
- Creatinine: 1.3 mg/dL
- AST: 20 IU/L
- ALT: 22 IU/L
- Sodium: 138 mEq/L
- Potassium: 4.9 mEq/L
- Calcium: 9.6 mg/dL
- Ejection fraction: 66%

If the attending physician is considering the addition of GluSense to this patient's medication regimen, which of the following is a contraindication for prescribing this medication?

(A) Allergy contraindication

(B) Cardiovascular contraindication

(C) Drug interaction contraindication

(D) Hepatic contraindication

(E) Renal contraindication

(F) There is no contraindication in this patient and the medication can be prescribed

The correct answer is C. You are being asked for the most likely reason to not prescribe this medication to a given patient. Therefore, you need to look for either an absolute or relative contraindication for prescribing this medication in the drug ad. The Contraindications section states that GluSense is contraindicated for "use with medications causing hyperkalemia." The patient is currently receiving enalapril and spironolactone. Both of these medications are associated with the development of hyperkalemia. Furthermore, the patient's potassium level is 4.9 mEq/L, which is at the high level of normal. The patient is likely to become hyperkalemic once starting this medication. Based on this information, a drug-drug interaction (choice C) between GluSense and both enalapril and spironolactone is the most likely contraindication for use of this medication in this patient. Choice C is correct and choice F is incorrect.

The patient has a history of anaphylaxis to the fluoroquinolone levofloxacin. Although GluSense is contraindicated for use in patients with a sulfonamide allergy, there is no allergy contraindication for using this medication in patients with a fluoroquinolone allergy (**choice A**).

The only cardiovascular contraindication (**choice B**) listed for GluSense is NYHA Class III or IV heart failure. This patient has a normal ejection fraction of 66% (normal 55-70%) so does not meet the cardiovascular contraindication criteria for this drug. Although the patient's past history of myocardial infarction predisposes him to heart failure, the patient currently does not have heart failure so there is no contraindication. However, there is a warning for use of

GluSense in patients with cardiovascular disease. As indicated, this patient has a past history of a myocardial infarction as well as hyperlipidemia and hypertension. Therefore, this medication should be used cautiously in this patient. If GluSense is prescribed, the patient should be monitored closely but there is no cardiovascular contraindication for the use of this drug in this patient.

The patient has normal hepatic function (AST: 20 IU/L (normal <35 IU/L) and ALT 22 IU/L (normal <35 IU/L)); hence, there is no hepatic contraindication for using GluSense in this patient (**choice D**).

The patient has normal renal function (creatinine: 1.3 mg/dL (normal 0.5-1.4 mg/dL)); hence, there is no renal contraindication for using GluSense in this patient (**choice E**).

Patient Safety and Quality Improvement

Clinical Applications of Patient Safety and Quality Improvement

24

PRINCIPLES OF PATIENT SAFETY

Case: Within the past 2 years, a major tertiary care referral hospital experiences separate cases of a blood transfusion reaction due to incompatibility, 2 inpatient falls leading to significant injury, a wrong-site surgery, and a medication-dosing error causing a patient death.

- What is the most probable single underlying cause behind these medical errors?

Systems failures due to the complexity of health care delivery

Health care is not a single system, but rather multiple systems which all interact. These clinical microsystems are defined as a group of clinicians and staff working together with a shared clinical purpose to provide health care for a population of patients. Individual health care organizations contain multiple microsystems which evolve over time. It is the complexity of these systems that predispose patients to harm from medical error.

Health care in the United States is capable of achieving incredible results for even the most severely ill patients. However, it does not do so reliably and consistently. Medical errors plague our health delivery systems. The Institute of Medicine (IOM) estimates that 44,000–98,000 patients die each year in the United States from preventable medical errors. This translates to more annual deaths than motor vehicles accidents, HIV, and breast cancer. In addition to the toll that this takes in the form of human suffering, medical errors also represent a significant source of inefficiency and increased cost in the health care system.

The causes of these adverse events are not usually from people intentionally seeking to harm patients, but rather from the complexity of the health care system together with the inherent capability for human error. The causes of these errors are varied, and can include failures made in administering medication, performing surgery, reporting lab results and making a diagnosis, to name a few. The most severe of these medical errors are referred to as **sentinel events.** A sentinel event is an adverse event in which death or serious harm to a patient has occurred; it usually refers to an event that is not at all expected or acceptable (e.g., operating on the wrong patient or body part, abduction of an infant from the hospital, patient suicide while admitted to the hospital). The choice of the word *sentinel* reflects the egregiousness of the injury (e.g., amputation of the wrong leg) and the likelihood that investigation of such an event will reveal serious problems in current policies or procedures.

It is unacceptable for patients to suffer preventable harm caused by a health care system whose purpose is to provide healing and comfort. Improving patient safety is the responsibility of every health care professional and requires a comprehensive team effort. Collectively, health care needs to learn from past errors and develop systems of care which prevent future errors from harming patients (e.g., process of root cause analysis).

Systems in health care delivery can be redesigned to **make it difficult for health care personnel to do the wrong thing** and **easier to consistently do the right thing**.

UNDERSTANDING MEDICAL ERROR

Classifications of Medical Errors

Medical errors can be classified as **errors of commission** (doing something wrong) or **errors of omission** (failing to do the right thing). Errors of omission are more difficult to recognize than errors of commission, but are thought to represent a larger percentage of medical errors.

Examples are ordering a medication for a patient with a documented allergy to that medication (**error of commission**), and failing to prescribe low-dose unfractionated heparin as venous thromboembolism prophylaxis for a patient undergoing hip replacement surgery (**error of omission**).

> Case: A 47-year-old man presents to the outpatient clinic with complaints of shoulder pain and is diagnosed with arthritis. The clinician treating him administers a shoulder corticosteroid injection without reviewing the patient's medication list prior to the procedure. The patient has been taking Coumadin for atrial fibrillation and develops hemarthrosis.

- Error classified as a lapse or omission

Lapses are missed actions or omissions (e.g., forgetting to monitor serum sodium in a patient undergoing diuresis for congestive heart failure). Lapses are not directly observable (i.e., you cannot directly 'see' a lack of memory). **Slips** are observed actions that are not carried out as intended (e.g., accidentally injecting a medication intravenously when it was meant to be given subcutaneously). **Mistakes** are a specific type of error brought about by a faulty plan or incorrect intentions; the intended action is wrong (e.g., barium swallow on a patient with suspected esophageal perforation or giving steroids to a patient with acute glaucoma).

The figure below clarifies the relationship further.

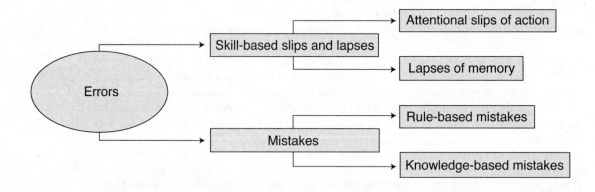

Case: After an unexpected 3-hour delay in the operating room due to a problem in the electrical system, an operating room team rushes to get started in order to complete the scheduled elective procedures. The team elects not to perform the mandatory sponge count at the end of the first surgery in order to get the next case started sooner. The patient returns 2 weeks later with abdominal pain and is found on x-ray to have a retained foreign object (a sponge) in the abdominal cavity.

- Error due to 'violation' in policy

Violations are conscious failures to adhere to procedures or regulation. Violations differ from slips, lapses and mistakes because they are deliberate actions, i.e., intentionally doing something against the rules. Reasons for violations may include time constraints, unfamiliarity with policy, or motivation by personal gain. A health care professional may consider that a violation is well-intentioned; however, if it results in an adverse event it would still technically constitute a 'violation' rather than an error.

Case: A 65-year-old man presents to the emergency department with sudden epigastric pain. He has a history of alcoholism, and the treating physician suspects a diagnosis of pancreatitis. Despite the fact that the patient denies alcohol use for several years, has normal blood levels of pancreatic enzymes, and has an abnormal EKG, he is treated for pancreatitis and the actual diagnosis of myocardial infarction is delayed.

- Error due to 'anchoring bias'

Anchoring bias describes when a clinician relies on and clings steadfastly to the initial diagnostic impression, despite subsequent information to the contrary. In many cases the features of a patient's presentation allow the clinician to make a correct initial diagnostic impression; however, in certain cases subsequent developments in the patient's course will prove inconsistent with the first impression. Anchoring bias refers to the tendency to hold on to the initial diagnosis, even in the face of disconfirming evidence.

Case: A 33-year-old woman with a breast lump is asked if it is tender. When she says that it is tender, the clinician confirms the suspected diagnosis of a cyst. No further history is obtained and the clinician fails to realize there has been an increase in size, associated adenopathy and fixation to the chest wall (hence the tenderness), all suggesting breast cancer.

- Error due to 'confirmation bias'

Confirmation bias may accompany anchoring, and refers to the tendency to focus on evidence that supports an initial diagnosis, rather than to look for evidence that refutes it or provides greater support to an alternative diagnosis.

Case: A 24-year-old sexually active woman is seen by her ob/gyn physician for complaints of abdominal pain. She is evaluated briefly and treated for a UTI without any other tests being performed. The next day, the patient presents to the emergency department and is diagnosed with a ruptured appendicitis.

- Error defined as **'premature closure'**

Premature closure is acceptance of a diagnosis before it has been fully vetted by considering alternative diagnoses or searching for data that contradict the initial diagnosis. In this case the physician finds a cause that fits the clinical picture and ceases to search for other diagnostic possibilities.

Case: A 4-week-old infant is brought to the emergency department by his parents after he develops an episode of emesis with an observed period of apnea. Three other infants were seen in the emergency department earlier this week with the flu. The infant is discharged home with instructions for flu management, but the parents return with him later, reporting that the child had another episode of apnea. The patient is further evaluated and subsequently transferred to the children's hospital with the clinical diagnosis of apnea from gastroesophageal reflux.

- Cognitive error classified as **'availability bias/heuristic'**

Availability bias/heuristic is the tendency to make the diagnosis of a current patient biased by recent or vividly recalled cases or events, rather than on prevalence or probability.

Case: During her third visit to an outpatient clinic for shortness of breath, a 57-year-old woman with documented pneumonia is treated with antibiotics and sent home. She later presents to the emergency department with exacerbation of dyspnea and is admitted to the medical service, where she is found to have hypoxia from heart failure.

- Error due to **'diagnosis momentum'**

Diagnosis momentum is a bias that occurs when the diagnosis considered by one clinician becomes a definitive diagnosis as it is passed from one clinician to the next; it then becomes accepted without question by clinicians down the line. It is the medical equivalent of "following the crowd."

Case: A patient with a known heroin addiction presents with abdominal pain. The treating physician assumes the pain to be a sign of opiate withdrawal and manages the patient accordingly with admission to the inpatient med-psychiatry ward. Later during the hospital stay the patient's pain increases and he develops peritonitis from a missed bowel perforation.

- Error related to **'framing effects'**

Framing effects: Diagnostic decision-making unduly biased by subtle cues and collateral information. This can lead to diagnostic error by allowing the way the story is framed to influence the diagnosis.

Human Factors that Cause/Influence Medical Errors

An understanding of medical error requires comprehension of the personal situations and factors associated with the risk of error. Human beings have limited memory and attention capacity. People can make errors when distracted or overtasked. The risk of error is exacerbated by conditions of fatigue, stress, and illness.

Case: A 9-year-old-boy is admitted to the pediatric oncology service for the treatment of a hemolytic malignancy, and is started on chemotherapy ordered from the pharmacy. The hospital pharmacist is working a double shift because 2 other pharmacists called in sick. The hospital is particularly busy and the pharmacist has not had a break all day. He accidentally sends the wrong dose of chemotherapy to the floor, after which the patient develops a hypotensive reaction. The patient is successfully resuscitated with fluids and supportive care.

- What contributed to this adverse patient event?

The risk of medical error is increased when health care professionals work under less than ideal circumstances, especially when well-designed safety systems are not in place. Poor working conditions include:

- Inexperience (especially when combined with lack of supervision)
- Time pressures
- Poor safety procedures (e.g., lack of staffing, lack of safety policies)
- Poorly designed human-equipment interfaces (e.g., difficult to program infusion pumps)
- Inadequate information (e.g., missing or outdated labs, illegible written orders, failure to communicate change in status, language barriers)

A helpful acronym which can be used by health care providers to assess their suitability to provide patient care is **IM SAFE**.

Illness

Medication

Stress

Alcohol

Fatigue

Emotion

The following actions have been demonstrated to limit errors caused by human factors.

- Avoid reliance on memory or vigilance.
- Simplify processes when possible.
- Standardize common procedures and processes.
- Routinely use checklists.

SYSTEMS-BASED PRACTICE

Lessons from high-reliability organizations (e.g., aviation, nuclear power plants) emphasize the importance of approaching errors on a **systems level** rather than a personal level with blame. It is easier to redesign the conditions under which people work than to attempt to change fallible human nature. When a system fails (i.e., medical error occurs), the immediate question should be **why did it fail**, not 'who caused it to fail.'

A classic example of a systems-based approach to patient safety is the removal of concentrated potassium from general hospital wards. This action was intended to prevent the inadvertent preparation of IV solutions with concentrated potassium, an error that had produced small but consistent numbers of deaths for many years. This particular approach is called a 'forcing function,' where the system is redesigned in a way that forces an individual to avoid making the error due to process design, rather than relying on individual memory. Think of a car that won't allow you to start the engine unless your foot is on the brake.

The "Swiss-cheese model of error" (James Reason, 1991) helps to identify the multiple factors that can often contribute to an error resulting in patient harm.

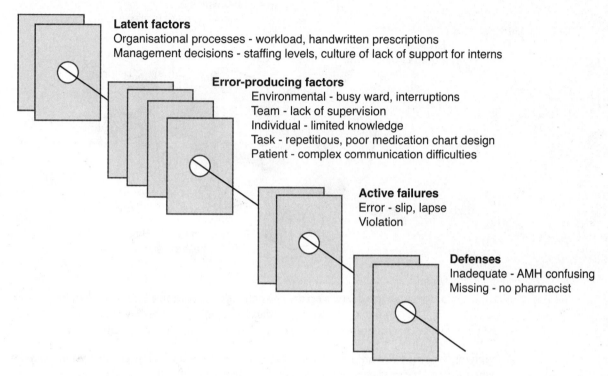

Latent factors
Organisational processes - workload, handwritten prescriptions
Management decisions - staffing levels, culture of lack of support for interns

Error-producing factors
Environmental - busy ward, interruptions
Team - lack of supervision
Individual - limited knowledge
Task - repetitive, poor medication chart design
Patient - complex communication difficulties

Active failures
Error - slip, lapse
Violation

Defenses
Inadequate - AMH confusing
Missing - no pharmacist

Source: James Reason, 1991

The layers represent barriers which prevent human error from causing patient harm. In a perfect world, these defenses would be impenetrable and patients would always be safe. In reality, these defenses have holes (hence, 'Swiss cheese'), which represent latent hazards (e.g., poor system design, lack of supervision, equipment defects). Occasionally the holes line up and a patient is injured.

Patient harm can be avoided by building systems with successive layers of protection (e.g., awareness, alarms, policies) and removal of latent errors (i.e., plug the holes).

Case: A 45-year-old man presents for treatment of acute sinusitis. He is prescribed antibiotics, after which he suffers a severe allergic reaction requiring hospitalization. Despite attempts of resuscitation, the patient sustains a cardiac arrest and dies. Later review of his medical record reveals a documented allergy to the antibiotic that was prescribed.

• How do we learn from this event to prevent a similar occurrence in the future?

An example of the "Swiss cheese model" follows below.

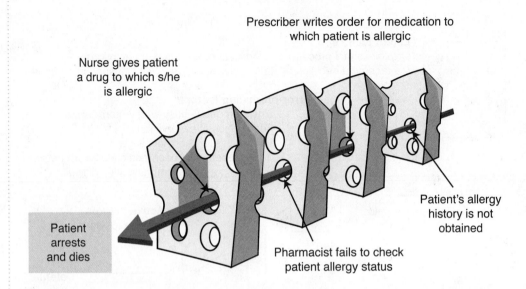

This example details a **medication error**. The patient's medication allergy is not obtained in the initial history, thus leading to the wrong medication being prescribed by the clinician, filled by the pharmacist, and administered by the nurse. The final result is the patient's death.

Applying 'systems-thinking' here, the question to be addressed is, "How can the system be redesigned so it is able to absorb the error before it reaches the patient?"

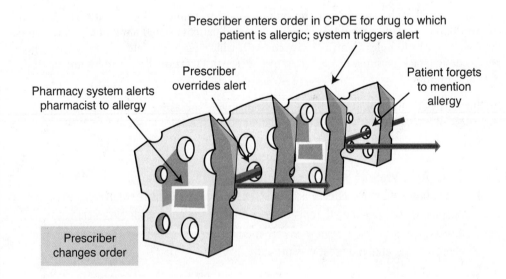

A systems-based redesign seeks not to *remove* the possibility of error, but rather to **create/reinforce barriers to harm**. For this case, one example would have been to implement a computer physician order entry (CPOE) based on the patient's electronic health record, which could have alerted the prescriber and pharmacist to the allergy.

Disclosure of Medical Errors

Known medical errors should be openly disclosed to the affected patient or, in certain circumstances, their families. During error disclosure, it is crucial to prepare the appropriate environment for disclosure. Be sure to arrange to have the proper time, place, and people involved, including arrangement of follow-up care and psychosocial support.

> Case: A 29-year-old man is brought to the emergency department after falling from a ladder. He is evaluated in the trauma bay and subsequently admitted to the hospital with a bilateral calcaneal fracture and stable L4/L5 compression fracture of the spine. The nurse notices that the blood pressure cuff used on the patient had blood stains on it from a prior patient treated for a motor vehicle collision. The prior patient was known to have hepatitis C. Somehow the cuff was not changed or cleaned before being used on the new patient, thus potentially exposing him to hepatitis C.
>
> • What information should be conveyed to the patient who was exposed?

An error disclosure should include the following 3 elements:

1. Accurate description of the events and their impact on the patient
2. Sincere apology showing care and compassion
3. Assurance that steps are being taken to prevent the event from happening in the future

Often the most senior physicians responsible for the patient and most familiar with the case will make the official disclosure.

QUALITY IMPROVEMENT PRINCIPLES

Only 5% of patient harm is directly due to individual incompetence or poor intentions. People need to be accountable, but system-based changes are needed to truly transform care. Blaming individuals and taking punitive actions for honest mistakes/errors do little to improve the overall safety of the health system. The most effective approach is to **find out how the error happened**, rather than who did it, and then **fix the system** to prevent a similar error from causing harm to patients in the future.

> Case: Two days after undergoing a hysterectomy for uterine fibroids, a woman is restarted on her outpatient dose of rivaroxaban (a new oral anticoagulant). The patient has a known history of deep venous thrombosis, for which she receives pain control via an epidural catheter. Before removal of the epidural catheter, the anesthesia intern on the pain service reviews the medication list for anticoagulants, yet does not realize that rivaroxaban is an anticoagulation agent. Five days after removal of the catheter, the patient develops an epidural hematoma and sustains paraplegia.

Clinical Pearl

Be aware of the **second victim** of medical error: the health care professionals involved in the adverse event. Studies report that these individuals often have strong feelings of self-doubt, self-disappointment, shame, and fear, and in fact directly blame themselves for the event.

Without the proper support, this can lead to significant depression, and in extreme cases, suicide. It is important to support colleagues who have been involved in medical error, and to seek counseling and support for yourself if you yourself have been involved. As much as possible, the goal is to learn from the error and move on.

- What should be done with the intern to improve safety in the future?

  Find out *how* the intern made this error (i.e., how the system allowed the error to occur and result in harm to the patient) and then fix the system to prevent a similar error from causing injury to patients in the future.

Error Reporting

Collecting data on medical errors is essential for improving patient care. Reporting errors provides this data and allows opportunities to improve care by learning from failures of the healthcare system. Error reporting is facilitated by

- Anonymous reporting
- A simple and easy-to-use system
- Timely feedback
- Absence of punitive actions

Note that while 'near misses' do not necessarily need to be disclosed to patients, they should be reported to the system so they can be studied and used to inform system changes. It is important to prevent what was a 'near miss' this time from potentially harming a patient in the future.

Root Cause Analysis

"Root cause analysis" (RCA) is a retrospective approach to studying errors. It allows a team to identify problems in the system or process of care. It should be conducted by a knowledgeable team (consisting of representatives from all the specialties/professions involved in the event), focus on systems/process analysis rather than individual performance, and identify potential improvements that can be made to reduce the chance of similar errors in the future.

Case: A 16-year-old patient comes to deliver her baby. During the process of her care, an infusion intended exclusively for the epidural route is connected instead to the peripheral IV line and infused by pump. Within minutes, the patient experiences cardiovascular collapse. A cesarean section results in the delivery of a healthy infant, but the medical team is unable to resuscitate the mother.

- Describe an effective approach to studying this error so that future cases of patient harm are prevented.

The fishbone diagram (also known as a 'Cause and Effect' or Ishikawa diagram) is used to explore all the potential causes that result in a poor outcome. An example is as follows:

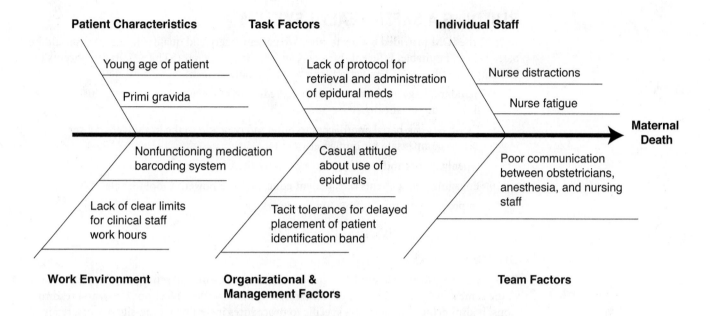

In the case presented here, systemic problems identified by the RCA would include medications being kept in the room, communication problems, inexperienced staff, and technology failures. Many solutions were then generated, including the removal of barriers to barcode scanning and changing the current medication ordering and dispensing policy. Another consideration would be to add a 'forcing function,' by redesigning the Luer lock on the epidural bag to be unable to connect to an IV line.

Failure Mode and Effects Analysis

The Failure Mode and Effects Analysis (FMEA) is a systematic tool that allows practitioners to anticipate what might go wrong with a device, product or process; determine the impact of that failure; and determine the likelihood of failure being detected before it occurs. Unlike the retrospective nature of RCA, the FMEA is a proactive approach to patient safety. It produces a risk priority number (RPN) based on the probability and relative impact of a failure.

$$\text{RPN} = \textbf{severity of the effect} \times \textbf{probability of occurrence of the cause} \times \textbf{probability of the detection}$$

For example: inadvertent esophageal intubation during elective surgery can severely affect patient outcome (rating of 10), but it has a low level of occurrence (2) and can be detected fairly easily (3).

Therefore, RPN for this failure mode = **10 x 2 x 3 = 60.**

BUILDING A SAFER HEALTH SYSTEM

In 2001 the IOM provided 6 aims to improve patient safety and quality; health care should be **S**afe, **T**imely, **E**quitable, **E**fficient, **E**ffective, and **P**atient-centered (STEEEP). Basic concepts for building a health care system which achieves these aims include:

- Standardizing care whenever possible, reducing reliance on memory (e.g., using checklists for important steps)
- Using systems-based approaches to build safety nets into the health care delivery process to compensate for human error
- Openly report and study errors (e.g., using RCA to learn from error)
- Engaging with patients (i.e., patient education is a powerful tool for safety)
- Improving communication and teamwork

Surgery

Patient safety in surgery is similar to patient safety in non-surgical settings, and involves many of the same issues including medication error, hospital-acquired infection (HAI), and readmissions. It also includes some errors specific to procedures including wrong-site surgery, retained foreign objects, and surgical site infections.

A **wrong-site procedure** is an operation or procedure done on the wrong part of the body or on the wrong person. It can also mean the wrong surgery or procedure was performed. Wrong-site procedures are rare and preventable, but they do still occur. Using a standard system of confirming the patient, site, and intended procedure with the medical team and patient before the procedure starts is a widely employed method of reducing or eliminating these types of errors.

> Case: A 59-year-old man with unresectable lung cancer presents to the emergency department with acute shortness of breath. A chest radiograph demonstrates a right sided malignant pleural effusion. The thoracic surgeon intending to drain the pleural effusion mistakenly places the chest tube on the left side after reading an x-ray of another patient. Post-procedure chest x-ray shows a persistent pleural effusion on the right lung. A second chest tube is then placed, this time in the patient's right chest. The patient remains stable and his breathing improves. The left chest tube is removed after confirmation that there is no air leak. There are no further sequelae.
>
> - How could this adverse event be prevented?

A team supported by the World Health Organization's "**Safe Surgery Saves Lives**" program designed a surgical safety checklist designed to improve team communication and consistency of care with the intent of reducing complications and deaths associated with surgery. The premise of the safe surgical checklist is that many common surgical complications are preventable. Implementation of the checklist was associated with significant reductions in the rates of death and complications including wrong-site surgery.

Among other benefits, the surgery checklist helps ensure appropriately administered antibiotic prophylaxis which reduces the incidence of surgical wound infection. The timing of antibiotic administration is critical to efficacy.

- The first dose should be given preferably within 30 minutes before incision.
- Re-dosing at 1 to 2 half-lives of the antibiotic is recommended for the duration of the procedure.
- In general, postoperative administration is not recommended.

Antibiotic selection is influenced by the organism most likely to cause a wound infection in the specific procedure.

Common Elements of Safe Surgery Checklist

- Confirm patient identity, planned procedure and marking of site
- Review patient allergies
- Ensure necessary equipment is present (e.g., pulse-oximetry)
- Introduce team members to each other
- Review critical steps of the procedure
- Address need for preoperative antibiotics
- Determine airway risk
- Determine estimated blood loss

Medications

Medication errors occur when a patient receives the wrong medication or where the patient receives the right medication but in the wrong dosage or manner (e.g., medication given orally instead of IV, or correct medication given at the wrong time). These errors represent one of the most common causes of preventable patient harm.

> Case: A 54-year-old woman (Susan Jones) is admitted to the hospital and diagnosed with metastatic breast cancer for which chemotherapy is administered. During her hospitalization she mistakenly receives an anticoagulation medication intended for the woman next to her in the room who has a similar name (Suzanne Jonas). The mistake is recognized after the first dose and the medication discontinued without any complications. Later during the same admission, she is inadvertently given an overdose of Dilaudid when the verbal order of 2 mg is administered intravenously instead of orally. She experiences lethargy and hypotension which resolve with supportive care during a brief stay in the ICU.
>
> - What are the risk factors contributing to the occurrence of these medication errors?

Several factors can increase the risk of medication errors:

- Inadequate confirmation of patient identity prior to medication administration
- Look-alike and sound-alike (rifampin/rifaximin) medications

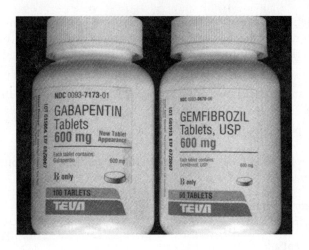

Look-alike Medications

- Illegible hand-written prescriptions/orders can result in a pharmacist or nurse administering the wrong drug or wrong dose of medication
- Use of certain abbreviations can result in misinterpretation of the order

The Joint Commission recently created a **"Do Not Use"** list of abbreviations for health professionals.

Official "Do Not Use" List[1]		
Do Not Use	*Potential Problem*	**Use Instead**
U, u (unit)	Mistaken for "0" (zero), the number "4" (four) or "cc"	Write "unit"
IU (International Unit)	Mistaken for IV (intravenous) or the number 10 (ten)	Write "International Unit"
Q.D., QD, q.d., qd (daily)	Mistaken for each other	Write "daily"
Q.O.D., QOD, q.o.d, qod (every other day)	Period after the Q mistaken for "I" and the "O" mistaken for "I"	Write "every other day"
Trailing zero (X.0 mg)* Lack of leading zero (.X mg)	Decimal point is missed	Write X mg Write 0.X mg
MS	Can mean morphine sulfate or magnesium sulfate	Write "morphine sulfate" Write "magnesium sulfate"
MSO4 and MgSO4	Confused for one another	

[1] Applies to all orders and all medication-related documentation that is handwritten (including free-text computer entry) or on pre-printed forms.

Source: jointcommission.org

The "**5R's**" describe a strategy used to help prevent medication error by confirming the following 5 items prior to administering any medication.

- Right drug
- Right patient
- Right dose
- Right route
- Right time

Performing **medication reconciliation** (a review of the patient's complete medication list during any transition of care) is also intended to prevent inadvertent inconsistencies in the medication regimen.

Other systems changes that have saved countless lives:

- Removal of high-risk medications from certain clinical settings
- 'Unit dose administration,' in which medications packaged in ready-to-use units are prepared by the pharmacy and delivered to the clinical floor (this practice has resulted in fewer medication errors compared with having nurses perform mixing and dispensing on the floor)

The **integration of information technology** has also helped to reduce medication errors. Studies have shown that Computerized Physician Order Entry (CPOE) is an effective means of reducing medication error. It involves entering medication orders directly into a computer system rather than on paper or verbally. CPOE can decrease prescribing errors by automatically alerting the prescriber or pharmacist to allergies, potential drug-drug interactions or an incorrect dose.

Other technologies that have been designed to improve medication errors include barcoding to confirm correct patient identity and smart-pumps to prevent inappropriate dosage of IV medications.

Infections

Hospital-acquired infections (HAI) can be avoided. They are preventable, adverse events which may be caused by failing to adhere to evidence-based prevention strategies. Common HAIs include UTI (most common 35-40%), hospital-acquired pneumonia/ventilator-acquired pneumonia (15-20%), surgical site infection (20%), and central line infection (10-15%).

Case: A 42-year-old man has surgery to repair a right inguinal hernia. His post-operative course is complicated by excessive post-op pain requiring IV narcotics. Ten hours after surgery he develops pubic pain. He has not voided since before surgery. A bedside ultrasound confirms a distended bladder indicating acute urinary retention. A urinary catheter is placed by a new nurse who is not familiar with sterile technique. The catheter immediately yields 800 cc of urine and the patient's pubic pain resolves. The patient requests to have the catheter left in place over the next 2 days. On post-operative day 3 the patient develops a fever to 101°C. A urine analysis and culture reveal an acute urinary infection.

- What steps can be taken to reduce the likelihood of this complication?

There are some common approaches which can help to reduce HAI:

- Hand washing
- Use of sterile technique
- Use of preoperative prophylactic antibiotics (SSI)
- Elevating the head of the bed (ventilation associated pneumonia)
- Limiting use and duration of indwelling urinary catheters (UTI)
- Following evidence-based protocols for central line placement
  - Hand washing prior to procedure
  - Wearing a cap, mask, sterile gown and gloves
  - Preparation of site with chlorhexidine
  - Use of sterile barrier
  - Removal of the line as soon as possible

Pressure Ulcers

Pressure, or decubitus, ulcers are often preventable. Approaches to avoid this complication include performing risk assessments to identify vulnerable patients (e.g. paraplegics, diabetics, malnutrition, immobility, etc.).

Case: A 65-year-old woman with type 2 diabetes and BMI 44 is being treated in the hospital for diabetic ketoacidosis. She has a urinary catheter in place to monitor urine output and does not get out of bed to go to the bathroom. She has refused ambulation or getting out of bed to a chair due to feeling very fatigued. Later during the hospital stay she develops a fever. Physical exam reveals a stage III infected decubitus ulcer over the sacral prominence.

- How could this complication have been prevented?

Preventive activities for high-risk patients include daily inspection of skin, appropriate skin care and minimizing pressure through frequent repositioning and use of pressure relieving surfaces (e.g., airbeds).

Patient Falls

Patient falls are a common cause of injury, both within and outside of health care settings. More than one-third of adults over 65 fall each year. Injuries can include bone fractures and head injury/intracranial bleeding, which both can lead to death.

Case: A 70-year-old woman is admitted to the nursing home after being treated in the hospital for a hip fracture sustained during a fall at home. She had an intramedullary nail placed and is currently able to ambulate with a walker. In addition to her hypertension medication, anxiolytic, dementia pills and a beta-blocker, she also takes post-operative pain medication every 4-6 hours. The patient was also placed on warfarin for DVT prophylaxis. On her way to the bathroom at night, she slips and falls, sustaining a head injury and significant intracranial hemorrhage.

- What steps can be taken to reduce the risk of serious injury from a fall?

Performing a fall risk assessment will help to select patients who can benefit from preventative resources (e.g. one-to-one observation, non-slip flooring, lowering the bed height). It is important to identify patients at high risk of sustaining serious injury from a fall. The following are known risk factors for patient fall:

- Advanced age (age >60)
- Muscle weakness
- Use of >4 prescription medications
- Impaired memory
- Difficulty walking (e.g., use of a cane or walker).

Unplanned Readmissions

Unplanned hospital readmissions following discharge are recognized as a serious cause of decreased quality and often result from complications or poor coordination of care. Improving communication, reinforcing patient education, and providing appropriate support to patients at risk for readmissions are all strategies to reduce unplanned readmissions.

Case: A 79-year-old patient is admitted to the cardiology service and treated for acute CHF. He is started on a new medication regimen including a diuretic which relieves his symptoms and improves his cardiac function. He is discharged home, though he returns to the hospital 10 days later with another episode of CHF. During the readmission, the team notices that the patient never filled his new prescriptions and was not taking the prescribed diuretic while at home.

- What actions can be taken to prevent this from happening again?

Recommendations to improve the discharge process and prevent readmissions are as follows:
- Provide timely access to care following a hospitalization
- Communicate and coordinate care plan with patients and other providers
- Improve the discharge planning and transition processes
- Ensure patient education and support to optimize home care

Teamwork

Providing safe health care relies on health care professionals working together as a team. Well-functioning teams deliver higher quality and safer care. The need for improved teamwork has led to the application of teamwork training principles, originally developed in aviation, to a variety of health care settings. Simple changes to behavior and culture have had a profound impact on the culture of teamwork and safety in patient care.

Case: A resident responds to a cardiac code 10 minutes late because he was not aware that he was on code-duty. Upon arrival the patient is actively having chest compressions performed by a physician assistant. A nurse brings in the cardiac arrest cart and a respiratory technician places on oxygen mask on the patient and begins bag-mask ventilation. The resident asks for a blood pressure and heart rate to be checked. The respiratory tech and physician assistant both attempt to find a pulse on the patient's wrist, interrupting chest compressions and ventilation. The nurse simultaneously lowers the bed to place electrodes for an ECG which makes the oxygen mask fall off to the floor. The ECG demonstrates ventricular fibrillation and the resident calls to "shock the patient." No one is certain how to work the defibrillator. The patient expires.

- How can teamwork be improved to achieve a better outcome during the next cardiac code?

Effective teams share the following characteristics:
- Common purpose/shared mental model
- Measurable goals
- Effective leadership
- Effective communication
- Mutual support
- Respect value of all team members

Briefs and **huddles** are effective tools for teamwork. The team *brief* is used for planning, and is a short 'time-out' prior to starting the delivery of care in order to discuss team formation, assign essential roles, establish expectations and climate, and anticipate outcomes and likely contingencies. The *huddle* is used for team problem-solving, and is performed on an ad hoc basis to reestablish situational awareness, reinforce plans already in place, and assess the need to adjust the plan.

Clinical Communication Skills

Communication failures have been identified as a root cause in the majority of serious patient safety events. Patient safety and quality in health care improve when physicians communicate effectively with colleagues, patients, and families. Several techniques have been developed to enhance clinical communication skills.

Case: A 25-year-old woman is admitted to the ICU following a motor vehicle collision, during which she sustained a significant head injury. She is intubated and monitored for increased ICP. The nurse coming on the night shift notices that the patient's pupils are dilated, and she is uncertain if this is a change in the patient's status. The nurse pages the resident on-call to see the patient. The resident evaluates the patient but does not speak with the nurse and is not aware of the nurse's concern of a change in status. No intervention is taken. The following morning during rounds the neurosurgical team finds the patient brain dead from herniation.

- How could communication be improved to prevent this error?

SBAR is a form of structured communication first developed for use in naval military procedures. It has been adapted for health care as a helpful technique used for communicating critical information that requires immediate attention and action concerning a patient's condition.

The following is an example of SBAR communication:

- **S**ituation: What is going on with the patient? "I am calling about Mr. Smith in room 432 who is complaining of shortness of breath."

- **B**ackground: What is the clinical background or context? "The patient is a 67-year-old man post-operative day one from a left total hip replacement. He has no previous history of pulmonary or cardiac disease."

- **A**ssessment: What do I think the problem is? "His breath sounds are decreased bilaterally and his oxygenation is only 87% on room air. He was getting IV Ringer's lactate at a rate of 150 cc/hour, in addition to 5 liters fluid replacement and 4 units of blood in the operating room. I would like to rule out acute pulmonary congestion from fluid overload."

- **R**ecommendation: What would I do to correct it or what action is being requested? "I've already started supplemental oxygen and I feel strongly that the patient should be assessed for pulmonary overload, his fluids stopped and potentially given a diuretic. Are you available to come in?"

Case: During resuscitation of a cardiac code, the physician running the code states that she thinks epinephrine should be given intravenously. The nurse is uncertain if this was an order and believes that the doctor may have been just thinking out loud. No epinephrine is given. The doctor mistakenly assumes that the drug was administered and that it was not effective in reviving the patient. Precious time is lost until it is realized that no medication has been given.

- What communication technique can be used to avoid this error?

A **call-out** is a strategy used to communicate important or critical information. The goals of a call-out are to inform all team members simultaneously during team events, help team members anticipate next steps, and help create a shared mental model.

Case: A hospital lab technician phones a nurse to inform him of a critical serum calcium value in one of his patients. The nurse mistakenly hears a different number and believes the calcium to be only mildly elevated. The patient develops a symptomatic arrhythmia and requires transfer to the ICU for further appropriate care.

- How can techniques in effective communication be used to prevent this error?

A **read-back or check-back** is a communication technique commonly used in the military and aviation industry, and is now increasingly employed in health care to guard against miscommunication. Safety organizations encourage health care professionals to make a routine practice of reading back verbal orders or critical labs to ensure accuracy.

Case: During a clinical rotation on the pediatric ICU, you are invited by the chief resident to observe the operative repair of a congenital heart lesion in the pediatric cardiac surgery operating room. When you arrive in the OR the patient is already intubated and anesthetized, and procedures are underway to prep the patient for surgery. During the start of the case you see that an operative team member inserts the urinary catheter with a clear breach in sterile technique. This is neither noticed by the team member inserting the catheter nor mentioned by anyone else in the room. Being new to this setting, you are unaware whether different practices for sterile insertion are used in pediatric patients.

- What would you do to address your concern?

Critical language is a form of assertive structured communication which provides key words that enable members of the team to speak when patient safety concerns arise. These key phrases are uniformly understood by all to mean "stop and listen to me; we have a potential problem."

The acronym **CUS** is used to remember these key words.
- "I'm <u>c</u>oncerned"
- "I'm <u>u</u>ncomfortable"
- "I think this is a <u>s</u>afety issue"

Speaking up for patient safety is the responsibility of every member of the health care team. It is important to speak up for the patient. It may be intimidating to speak up when you are the most junior member of the team and at times uncertain if a safety issue is actually in question; however, as people with the privilege of caring for others, health care workers have to value our responsibility to the patient above all else. **Speak up if you witness an error or the potential for an error**. Make sure to report adverse events so others can study and learn from them—informing system-based approaches to improving patient safety.

Handoffs

Errors during handoffs and sign-outs can be mitigated by ensuring an accurate and effective transfer of pertinent patient information to the receiving health care professional. This has immediate applications to on-call sign-outs and changes of shift, but it also affects other scenarios such as hospital- and unit-floor-transfers.

> Case: A diabetic patient with an ankle fracture is signed-out to the covering intern from a team member in a hurry to leave the hospital. Later that night the patient develops sinus tachycardia thought be related to pain, and the covering intern orders more pain medication. Unknown to the covering intern, the patient was found earlier to have an incidental pulmonary embolism. This information was forgotten during the hurried sign-out. The patient develops chest pain, dyspnea and ultimately dies from progression of the PE.
>
> • How can this adverse event be avoided in the future?

An effective handoff encompasses the following principles:
- Active process
- Prioritize sick patients
- Verbal + written
- Have a set system
- Limit distractions
- Allow sufficient time
- Ensure updated information

Quality Improvement Roadmap

The methods used to approach quality and process improvement are as follows:
1. Identify the problem.
2. Measure the problem.
3. Organize a team.
4. Flowchart the process.
5. Develop a range of interventions to fix the problem.
6. Measure the impact of the interventions.

Case: A hospital is interested in reducing the number of medication errors in the inpatient geriatric unit. The current medication ordering system has been in place for 15 years and consists of written orders on slips of paper being sent to pharmacy by pneumatic tubes, and then receiving the medication in a batched collection system on the unit. Nurses are required to then sort through the batched medications to identify the correct one for their patient(s). Over the past year, the severity of the admitted geriatric patients has increased, along with the number of medications required. There have been reports of possible increased rates of medication errors over the past 6 months.

- How will you approach improving the current process?

The following tools are commonly used in quality improvement:

Flow chart: map of all the steps in the current clinical process being evaluated
- Flow charting a process helps the team clearly see the complexity of the process and the opportunities for improvement.

Pareto analysis: process of rank-ordering quality improvement opportunities to determine which of the various potential opportunities should be approached first

Run chart (time plot): graphical record of a quality characteristic measured over time
- Run charts help the team determine if a change is a true improvement over time or just a random fluctuation.
  - A trend is defined as ≥5 consecutive points constantly increasing or constantly decreasing. If a trend is detected, it might indicate a non-random pattern that should be investigated.
  - A shift is a run containing ≥6 data points all above or all below the median and indicates a non-random pattern that should be investigated.

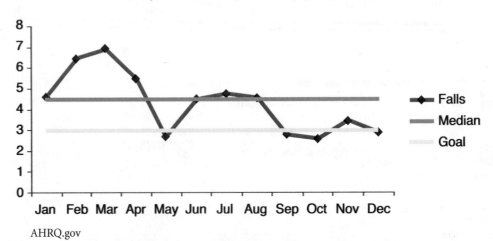

Sample Run Chart Plotting Patient Falls

Control chart: method used to distinguish between variations in a process due to common causes and those due to special causes. It is constructed by obtaining measurements of some characteristic of a process, summarizing with an appropriate statistic, and grouping the data by time period, location, or other process variables.

- Common cause variation is an inherent part of every process. It is random and due to natural or ordinary fluctuations in the system.

- Reducing variation improves the predictability of outcomes and helps reduce the frequency of adverse outcomes for patients.

- Special cause variation is due to irregular or unnatural causes that are neither predictable nor inherent to the process. Special cause variation should be identified and eliminated before making QI changes to a process.

There are many different types of control charts, depending on the statistic analyzed on the chart.

Interventions can take many forms, including automation, standardized process, and checklists. A forcing function is a very effective intervention for patient safety, as it does not rely on human memory or vigilance. A forcing function is an aspect of a design that prevents a target action from being performed. Examples are:

- Computer system that does not allow a drug to be ordered at a dose outside known safety parameters

- Enteral tubing designed to prevents accidental connections with IV ports

Measurements of quality include structure, process, outcomes, and balancing measures.

- **Structure** refers to equipment, resources, or infrastructure (e.g., number of ICU beds, certified infectious disease specialist on staff, ratio of nurses to patients)

- **Process measures** relate to an action involved in the care of patients that is believed to be associated with a particular outcome (e.g., use of preoperative antibiotics to reduce surgical site infections, using 2 means of patient identification prior to blood transfusion).

  - Typically easier to measure than outcome measures, and often serve as surrogates to outcomes

- **Outcome measures** reflect results related directly to the patient (e.g., survival, infection rates, number of admissions for heart failure)

- **Balancing measures** monitor for unintended consequences of a change or intervention made to a process or system. Some well-intended interventions can create unanticipated negative results in quality and safety.

  - For example, alarms have been placed on a number of medical devices and equipment to alert for problems (e.g., oxygen saturation falling below a set level). One negative result has been 'alarm fatigue.' Studies indicate that 85-99% of hospital alarms do not require clinical attention, but failure to respond to the rare critical alarm has resulted in patient death. This is a type of 'boy who cried wolf' phenomenon, where the frequency and prevalence of hospital alarms reduces our attention to them. Strategies are in place to customize alarms to alleviate some of the problem.

Quality models are specific techniques used in improving patient care.

PDSA (plan-do-study-act) refers to a rapid cycle of activities involved in achieving process or system improvement. It is a form of trial and error and consists of planning an intervention, trying it out (i.e. small scale pilot), observing results (e.g. data collection of quality measures), and acting on what is learned (e.g. implement change system-wide or go back to the planning stage with a new intervention).

Six Sigma is a data-driven, patient-centered approach focused on reducing variability. This organized and systematic method for strategic process improvement uses a step-by-step DMAIC method.

- **Define**: define the problem
- **Measure**: measure key quality metric
- **Analyze**: identify root causes
- **Improve**: determine optimal solutions
- **Control**: strive for sustainability of implemented change

Lean process focuses on removing waste from the process or system and adopting a value-added philosophy of patient care. Value-stream maps are created to optimize activities that add value from the patient point-of-view and remove activities that do not.

The following are steps that any health care practitioner can apply to improve safety and quality for patients.

- Follow safety protocols (e.g., hand washing)
- Speak up when there are safety concerns (e.g., medical errors and near misses)
- Practice good communication skills (e.g., SBAR)
- Educate patients about their care
- Take care of yourself (e.g., get appropriate sleep and control stress)
- Practice patient-centered care/recognize opportunities to enhance value for patients

CARE WELL DONE

The case below describes the incredible potential of the health care system. Applying the principles of patient safety and quality improvement to clinical care will enable health care to move closer to the goal of getting it right for every patient, every time.

> A 3-year-old girl falls into an icy fishpond in a small Austrian town in the Alps. She is lost beneath the surface for 30 minutes before her parents find her on the pond bottom and pull her up. CPR is started immediately by the parents on instruction from an emergency physician over the phone, and EMS arrives within 8 minutes. The girl has a body temperature of 36° C and no pulse. Her pupils are dilated and do not react to light. A helicopter takes the patient to a nearby hospital, where she is wheeled directly to an operating room. A surgical team puts her on a heart-lung bypass machine, her body temperature increases almost 10 degrees, and her heart begins to beat. Over the next few days her body temperature continues to rise to normal and her organs start to recover. While she suffered extensive neurologic deficits during this event, by age 5 with the help of extensive outpatient therapy, she recovers completely and is like any other little girl her age.

CHAPTER SUMMARY

- Medical errors result from the complexity of health care combined with the reality of human failure. Although accountability and responsibility are important, simply blaming people for errors they did not intend to commit does not address underlying failures in the system and is an ineffective way of improving safety.

- System-based redesigns in health care delivery are required and hold the greatest potential for advancing patient safety and quality improvement.

- Improving communication, teamwork and the culture of safety are effective methods in improving patient safety.

- Safety is a team effort requiring everyone on the care team to work in partnership with one another and with patients and families.

High Yield Facts

- Systems-based approaches to improving health care are superior to individual-level efforts or blame

- Preoperative checklists can prevent perioperative complications and safety events

- Evidence-based bundles (protocols) prevent central line infection

- Limiting the duration of urinary catheters decreased hospital acquired infections

- Head-of-bed elevation and oral care prevents ventilator associate pneumonia

- Medication reconciliation helps to prevent medication errors during transitions

- Hand hygiene is an important component of infection control

- Avoid the use of hazardous abbreviations

- Computerized physician order entry helps improve medication safety

- Identification of high risk patients is a key step in fall prevention

- Team training and communication can improve quality and safety

Practice Questions

1. A 36-year-old woman with HIV/AIDS and B-cell lymphoma is hospitalized for *Clostridium difficile*–associated diarrhea. Following treatment, the patient is discharged home with a prescription for a 14-day course of oral vancomycin. She is unable to fill the prescription at her local pharmacy because of a problem with her insurance coverage. While awaiting coverage approval, she receives no treatment. Her symptoms soon return, prompting an emergency department visit where she is diagnosed with toxic megacolon. Which of the following should be addressed in order to bring about changes that improve patient safety?

   (A) Prescribing physician

   (B) Pharmacist

   (C) Insurance company

   (D) Patient

   (E) Discontinuity of care

The answer is E. The main failure in this case occurred upon transition of care from the hospital to home. Addressing the discontinuities in care which arise at the time of transition has the greatest potential to improve patient safety.

Rather than dispensing blame to any of the parties involved in the error (**choices A–D**), focus should be given to implementing systems-based transformations to support patients during a transition (e.g. post-discharge telephone follow-up to identify and resolve potential medication issues early).

2. A 23-year-old man with a history of depression is admitted to the inpatient psychiatry ward after his third attempt at suicide with an intentional drug overdose. The patient is stabilized medically; however, he is put under 24-hour monitoring by the nursing staff due to repeated attempts at self-harm. During a change of shift, there is a mistake in communication and no one is assigned to the patient. The mistake is noticed 15 minutes into the new shift, and a member of the nursing team is assigned to watch the patient. Fortunately, during that 15-minute period, the patient made no attempt to harm himself. Which of the following statements is correct about this event?

   (A) This is a sentinel event and should be reported to the medical board.

   (B) This is a sentinel event and should be reported to the hospital and family.

   (C) This is a near-miss and should be reported to the hospital.

   (D) This is a near-miss and should be reported to the patient and family.

   (E) This is a near-miss and no reporting is required since the patient was not harmed.

The answer is C. The event described is a near-miss; there was an error which fortunately did not result in patient harm. Most near-misses need not be disclosed to patients or families (**choice D**), but they should be reported to the hospital so that the error can be studied and thus prevented in the future. A sentinel event (**choices A and B**) is an adverse event resulting in serious or permanent injury to a patient.

3. An 85-year-old woman is being transferred to an acute rehabilitation facility following a hospital admission for hip replacement surgery. Postoperatively during her hospital stay, she is started on deep vein thrombosis (DVT) prophylaxis medication with plans to continue the medication upon discharge. The intern and nurse who are discharging the patient fail to convey this new medication to the receiving treatment team at the rehabilitation center. The patient is not continued on her anticoagulation medication and sustains a DVT, leading to a fatal pulmonary embolus 3 weeks after transfer. Which of the following actions will facilitate quality improvement and the prevention of a similar error in the future?

(A) Determine which staff member(s) failed to order the medication

(B) Develop a process to increase the use of medication reconciliation

(C) Send a memo to all staff about the importance of DVT prophylaxis

(D) Educate patients about the dangers of DVT following hip surgery

(E) Conduct monthly audits to monitor medication errors at transitions of care

The answer is B. The goal of quality improvement (QI) is to achieve improvement by measuring the current status of care and then developing systems-based approaches to making things better. It involves both prospective and retrospective reviews and specifically attempts to avoid attributing blame. QI seeks to create systems to prevent errors from happening. In this case, developing a process to increase the use of medication reconciliation would be following the principles of QI. The other interventions in the answer choices are QA-based and/or simply not as effective in creating and sustaining a positive change. Quality assurance (QA) is an older term describing a process that is reactive and retrospective in nature; it is a form of 'policing' to ensure that quality standards have been followed. It often relies on audits and traditionally has focused on punitive actions for failures in quality, i.e., determining who was at fault after something goes wrong. QA has not proven to be very effective in transforming care.

Population Health Management 25

DEFINING POPULATION HEALTH

What is population health?

Case example: A 65-year-old woman presents to the emergency department at 3:00 AM with the acute onset of an asthma attack. She is treated with steroids and nebulizer treatments to stabilize her respiratory status. This is the third such presentation in the past 9 months. During her course of treatment it becomes evident that the patient is not able to get time off from work to see her primary care physician during clinic hours, did not receive an influenza vaccination this year, and continues to smoke 1 pack of cigarettes per day.

- What day-to-day factors are present which impact this patient's health outcomes with asthma?

- How would you to help to optimize her long-term management of asthma?

Health care in the United States has traditionally focused on the management of acute medical problems such as trauma, myocardial infarction, and stroke. Incredible advances have been made in these areas and outcomes from acute presentation of disease have steadily improved over the years, with outcomes among some of the best observed in any health system in the world.

However, the health care system here has lagged significantly in the area of disease prevention and health maintenance. Major disparities in access to preventative care services such as pre-natal care, cancer screening and diabetes management; together with social inequalities with respect to patient education and income; as well as persistent individual behaviors such as poor diet, lack of exercise and cigarette smoking have contributed to the very poor overall health status observed in the United States.

BIG GEMS (mnemonic for determinants of health)
- Behavior
- Income
- Genetics

- Geography
- Environment
- Medical care
- Social-cultural

Problems with patient safety and variations in care that do not follow evidence-based standards further erode the value of patient care. Ironically, the United States spends more on health care than any other nation in the world, yet ranks among the lowest in health measures, compared to other developed nations. Furthermore, the current rate of health care spending in the United States is unsustainable.

Population health is an approach to health care which addresses both individual and public health concerns in order to achieve optimal patient results. It is an approach to patient care which understands that health is influenced by several factors outside of traditional health care delivery models, including (but not limited to) social, economic, and environmental factors.

Population health management is fundamental to the transformation of health care delivery. Its principles recognize the importance of focusing attention not only on improving individual patient care, but also on improving the health of an entire population. In fact, direct health care accounts for only a small proportion of premature deaths in the United States.

- For example, the leading causes of premature death—smoking (435,000 deaths/year), obesity (400,000 deaths/year), and alcohol abuse (85,000 deaths/year)—are all preventable through interventions driven by population health management.

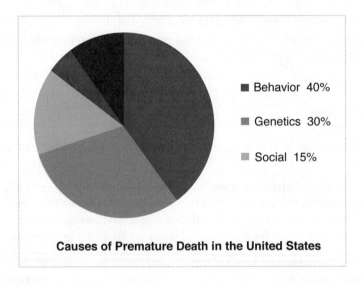

Causes of Premature Death in the United States

Population health management is, in effect, about coordinating care and improving access in order to enhance patient/family engagement and reduce variation in care to achieve better long-term outcomes at a reduced cost. The Institute for Healthcare Improvement (IHI) lists improving the health of the population as one of the 3 dimensions of its Triple Aim approach to optimizing health system performance.

IHI Triple Aim:
- Improve the patient experience of care (including quality and satisfaction)
- **Improve the health of populations**
- Reduce the per capita cost of health care

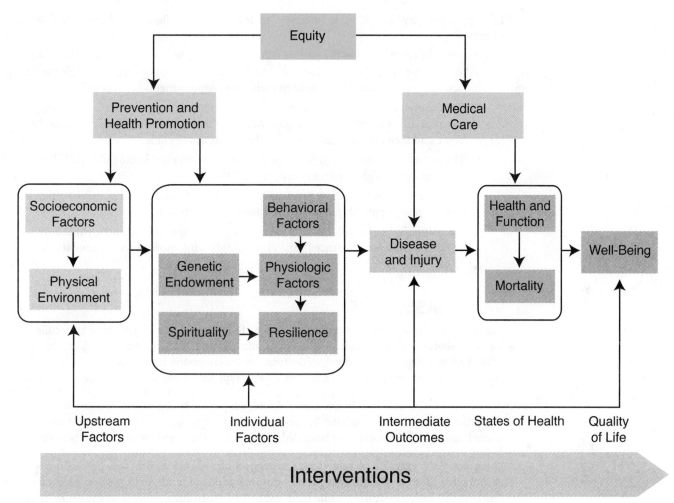

Source: Adapted from Stiefel M. Nolan KA. Guide to Measuring the Triple Aim: Population Health, Experience of Care, and Per Capita Cost. IHI Innovation Series white paper.Cambridge, Massachusetts: Institute for Healthcare Improvement; 2012. (Available on www.IHI.org)

IHI Population Health Composite Model

Population health management focuses on high-risk patients who are responsible for the majority of health care utilization while simultaneously addressing preventative and chronic care needs of the entire population. One of the first steps in this process is to define the target population (e.g., a hospital or clinic's entire service area or any subset, whether economic, geographic or demographic, or individuals with certain health conditions). Another important step is to identify the specific health status and needs of that group and deploy interventions and prevention strategies to improve the health of the group. The interventions target individuals, but they affect the entire population.

The incorporation of technology (e.g., electronic health records) and innovations in health care (e.g., digital home health monitoring) provide the infrastructure to support efforts in successful population health management. A key factor for the success of population health programs is automation, as managing populations can be highly complex. Technology-enabled solutions are essential to the efficient management of a program.

Let's say a primary care clinic is interested in improving population health for its diabetic patients.

- First, the clinic analyzes the patient registry generated by its electronic health records to identify high-risk type 2 diabetic patients who are not compliant with their medication and who frequently fail to keep their clinic appointments.

- Next, those patients are offered enrollment in a home hemoglobin A1C monitoring program, using a system which digitally records hemoglobin A1C levels taken in the home and then electronically transfers the results to the clinic.

- The system sends an alert to the clinical team when patients' hemoglobin A1C levels are consistently higher than a predetermined threshold.

- A nurse coordinator contacts these patients by phone to help manage medication compliance, answer patient questions, and encourage timely follow-up with clinic visits.

- A nutritionist works with patients to encourage healthy dietary choices, while a social worker addresses any financial constraints to following medical recommendations.

VALUE-BASED CARE

The traditional health care system operates under a **fee-for-service model**, where a fee is collected for each provision of health care service. For example, hospitals and physicians collect a fee each time a patient comes to the hospital for the treatment of congestive heart failure (CHF), including any diagnostic tests or procedures (e.g. chest x-ray, B-type natriuretic peptide, cardiac angiogram).

A new model of health care in the United States, supported by legislation, is accountable care. Under the Accountable Care Act, the fee-for-service model is being replaced with **value-based care**, where health care professionals are rewarded for keeping entire populations of patients healthy.

Using the CHF example, a value-based system would reward health care professionals for encouraging lifestyle changes that prevent hospital admissions for CHF, such as promoting a heart healthy diet, monitoring home fluid intake, and motivating patients to engage in regular exercise. Instead of rewarding exclusively for the treatment of acute medical problems, the new system provides incentives for the health care system to maintain healthy populations, prevent disease, and avoid acute medical problems through the active monitoring and management of chronic disease. **Quality in health care is measured by outcomes achieved**, rather than the *volume* of services delivered.

Note: Value in patient care can be defined as quality of care divided by total cost of care.

Strategies that increase quality and reduce unnecessary costs result in improved value for patients. Unnecessary costs may be generated from the following examples:

- Duplication of services (e.g., a surgeon orders a routine pre-operative ECG for a patient undergoing elective surgery, not realizing the same test was done 1 week ago in the primary care physician's office and was normal)

- Non evidence-based care (e.g., ordering antibiotics for a viral infection)

- Avoidable inefficiencies in care (e.g., a patient returns to the hospital with acute CHF 1 week after being treated for the same condition because he was unaware that a new diuretic had been started in the hospital and was therefore never filled upon discharge)

Failures in preventive health also lead to avoidable health care spending, as in hospitalization for the treatment of acute pneumonia in a patent who did not receive an influenza vaccination. Shifting the focus from volume of care to value of care will improve the overall status of health care in the United States and contain the currently unsustainable costs of care.

It is important **not to confuse value-based care** with **rationing of care**, which seeks to reduce needed services in order to preserve resources. Value-based care seeks to reduce unnecessary or unwanted waste in care which increases cost without increasing quality of care to the patient.

- Studies, for instance, have shown that performing stress cardiac imaging or advanced non-invasive imaging in patients without symptoms on a serial or scheduled pattern (e.g., every 1–2 years or at a heart procedure anniversary) rarely results in any meaningful change in patient management. This practice may, in fact, lead to unnecessary invasive procedures and excess radiation exposure without any proven impact on patients' outcomes.
  - An exception to this rule would be for patients >5 years after a bypass operation.
- Similarly, using antibiotics for a sore throat or runny nose that is due to a viral infection not only provides no immediate benefit to the patient, it may also increase harm from adverse drug reactions or development of antibiotic resistant bacterial strains.

Many health care organizations are developing guidelines and recommendations to promote value-based care. These approaches motivate patients and their clinicians to follow effective care practices and guide them away from unnecessary and ineffective care; the result is greater value and effectiveness of healthcare utilization. For example, Choosing Wisely™ (choosingwisely.org) is a national initiative of the American Board of Internal Medicine Foundation which promotes conversations between patients and physicians about unnecessary medical tests/procedures that increase cost without enhancing patient outcomes.

Population health management employs value-based care principles by promoting preventive care, encouraging care patterns that have been proven effective, and reducing waste and unnecessary care.

Value equation in health care:

$$\uparrow value = \frac{\uparrow quality}{\downarrow cost}$$

IMPLEMENTATION OF POPULATION HEALTH MANAGEMENT

The goal of population health management is to keep a patient population as healthy as possible. The components required to achieve this goal include the following:

- Delivery of patient care through multidisciplinary teams
- Coordination of care across care settings
- Increased access to primary care
- Patient education in disease self-management
- Emphasis on health behaviors and lifestyle choices
- Meaningful use of health information technology for data analysis, clinical communication, and outcome measurement

This requires clinicians to identify target populations of patients who may benefit from additional services, such as patients who require reminders for preventative care appointments or patients not meeting management goals. Continual access to patient data and analysis of outcomes is the key to providing proactive, preventive care.

Steps in Population Health Management:

Step 1: Define population

Step 2: Identify care gaps

Step 3: Stratify risks

Step 4: Engage patients

Step 5: Manage care

Step 6: Measure outcomes

Several advances in technology are required to perform effective population health management and accomplish risk stratification; identify gaps in care; achieve patient education, compliance education, disease state monitoring; ensure general wellness; as well as to implement and assess specific interventions targeted to selected populations.

- The electronic health record can produce integrated, accessible population-wide data systems capable of generating reports that drive effective quality and care management processes.
- Web-based tools designed to educate patients about their condition, promote self-care, and encourage preventative behaviors have been used successfully to reduce hospitalization rates by enabling patients to take charge of their health.
- Telemedicine programs have been implemented to establish remote care in order to facilitate patient outreach, allow patient follow-up after discharge from the hospital, and improve health care in rural populations.
- The automation of processes and programs is essential in order to make population health management feasible, scalable, and sustainable, such as a health IT system which targets patients in greatest need of services, generates alerts to those patients seeking appropriate and timely appointments with clinicians, and alerts clinicians in real-time to patient care needs.

However, technology alone will not be sufficient for population health management; effective **teamwork** in patient care is also important. Effective population health involves establishing multidisciplinary care teams to coordinate care throughout the entire continuum of care. High-performance clinical care teams can manage a greater number of patients and more comprehensively respond to patient care needs compared with individual clinicians working in isolation. Care teams can include physicians, nurses, nurse practitioners, physician assistants, pharmacists, patient navigators, medical assistants, dieticians, physical therapists, social workers, and care managers, and others.

The **patient-centered medical home (PCMH)** is one emerging model used to deliver patient-centered, value-based care, and it plays an important role in population health management. The medical home model emphasizes care coordination and communication beyond episodic care in order to transform primary care. It stresses prevention, early intervention and close partnerships with patients to tightly manage chronic conditions and maintain health. The PCMH is not necessarily a physical place, but rather an organizational model that delivers the core functions of primary health care. Key principles in this model include:

- Access to a personal physician who leads the care team within a medical practice
- Adoption of a whole-person orientation to providing patient care
- Integrated and coordinated care
- Focus on quality and safety

The medical home is intended to result in more personalized, coordinated, effective and efficient care. Many of the goals of PCMH directly support efforts in population health.

In 2006, the Massachusetts General Hospital (MGH) worked with the U.S. Centers for Medicare and Medicaid to establish 1 of 6 population health demonstration projects nationwide. During the 3-year demonstration, the MGH implemented strategies to improve health care delivery to its most vulnerable high risk patients—those with multiple health conditions and chronic disease. The hospital system took steps to address the needs of 2,500 of their highest-risk patients.

- Each patient was assigned to a comprehensive care team consisting of a primary care physician, experienced nurse case manager, social worker, and pharmacist.
- A non-clinical community resource specialist was employed to work with the care teams in addressing non-clinical factors influencing health outcomes (for example, if the patient was not able to come to the primary care office for a scheduled visit because of transportation issues, this specialist connected the patient to local transportation resources).

This structure of care allowed clinicians to focus the majority of their time on patients' medical needs. The results revealed a decrease in hospital readmissions by 20%, and a decrease in emergency room visits by 13% for the patients enrolled in the program. Satisfaction was extremely high among both patients and caregivers, and the system was associated with significant cost-savings. This is one example of using population health to increase quality while decreasing costs, thereby increasing value in patient care.

CHAPTER SUMMARY

- Population health management is an important strategy for improving the quality of patient outcomes, containing costs, and promoting health maintenance.

- Successful population health management requires data-driven clinical decision-making, transformations in primary care leadership, meaningful use of health technology and patient-family engagement.

- Accountable care involves an integrated, proactive approach to improving the quality of health in identified patient populations.

High Yield Topics

- Understanding and managing population risk (e.g., identifying care gaps)
- Care teams coordinating home health between clinic visits as well as during clinic encounters
- Informatics: sharing information seamlessly with EHR and patient portals
- Engaging patients in health maintenance: screening, prevention and behavioral health
- Measuring outcomes
- Reducing waste in the system (e.g., duplication, non-value added interventions)
- Improving chronic care: keeping patients out of hospital (optimize home and outpatient care)

KEY DEFINITIONS

- **Care cycle:** array of health services and care settings which address health promotion, disease prevention, and the diagnosis, treatment, management, and rehabilitation of disease, injury, and disability

- **Clinical care pathway:** integrated, multidisciplinary outline of anticipated care placed in an appropriate timeframe to help patients with a specific condition/set of symptoms move progressively through a clinical experience to positive outcomes

- **Clinical outcome:** end result of a medical intervention, such as survival or improved health

- **Clinical variation:** variation in the utilization of health care services that cannot be explained by variation in patient illness or patient preferences (Wennberg JH 2010)

- **Continuum of care:** concept involving an integrated system of care which guides and tracks patients over time through a comprehensive array of health services spanning all levels of intensity of care

- **Cost-effectiveness analysis:** analytic tool in which the costs and effects of at least 1 alternative are calculated and presented, as in a ratio of incremental cost to incremental effect; the effects are health outcomes (e.g., cases of disease prevented, years of life gained, or quality-adjusted life years) rather than monetary measures (e.g., cost-benefit analysis) (Gold et al. 1996)

- **Evidenced-based medicine**: applying the best available research results (evidence) when making decisions about health care
  - Health care professionals who perform evidence-based practice use research evidence, along with clinical expertise and patient preferences. Systematic reviews (summaries of health care research results) provide information which aids in the process of evidence-based practice.
    - For example, a health care provider recommends acetaminophen to treat arthritis pain in a patient who has recently had stomach bleeding. The health care provider makes this recommendation because research shows that acetaminophen is associated with less risk for stomach bleeds than other common pain relievers. The health care provider's recommendation is an example of evidence-based practice.
- **Health**: a state of complete physical, mental and social well-being, and not merely the absence of disease or infirmity (WHO definition)
- **Health inequity**: those inequalities in health deemed to be unfair or to stem from some form of injustice; the dimensions of being avoidable or unnecessary have often been added to this concept (Kawachi, Subramanian, and Almeida-Filho 2002)
- **Health-related quality of life**: impact of the health aspects of an individual's life on his quality of life or overall well-being (Gold et al. 1996)
- **Intervention**: any type of treatment, preventive care, or test that a person could take or undergo to improve health or to help with a particular problem
  - Health care interventions include drugs (prescription drugs or drugs that can be bought without a prescription), foods, supplements (such as vitamins), vaccinations, screening tests (to rule out a certain disease), exercises (to improve fitness), hospital treatment, and certain kinds of care (such as physical therapy).
- **Life expectancy**: average amount of time a person will live after a certain starting point, such as birth or the diagnosis of a disease
  - The calculation is based on statistical information comparing people with similar characteristics, such as age, gender, ethnicity, and health. In the United States, for example, the life expectancy from birth for men and women combined is 78.1 years. In England, it is 78.7, and in China it is 72.9 years.
- **Patient-centered**: approach to patient care that focuses on the priorities, preferences, and best interests of the patient
  - It is a partnership among practitioners, patients, and their families to ensure that (a) decisions respect patients' wants, needs, and preferences, and (b) patients have the education and support needed to make decisions and participate in their own care.
- **Patient centered medical home**: care delivery model whereby patient treatment is coordinated through the primary care physician to ensure that the patient receives the necessary care when and where she needs it, in a manner she can understand
  - The goal is to have a centralized setting which facilitates partnerships between individual patients, their personal physician, and when appropriate, their family. Care is facilitated by registries, information technology, health information exchange, and other means to assure that patients get optimal care.

- **Population:** any group of individuals for whom consideration of health or health care at the level of the group is likely to advance health

- **Population health:** health of a population as measured by health status indicators, and as influenced by social, economic, and physical environments; personal health practices; individual capacity and coping skills; human biology; early childhood development; and health services (Dunn and Hayes 1999)

- **Public health:** activities that a society undertakes to assure the conditions in which people can be healthy; these include organized community efforts to prevent, identify, and counter threats to the health of the public (Turnock 2004)

- **Quality of life:** a broad construct reflecting a subjective or objective judgment concerning all aspects of an individual's existence, including health, economic, political, cultural, environmental, aesthetic, and spiritual aspects (Gold, Stevenson, and Fryback 2002)

- **Quality measure:** clinical quality measures (CQMs) are a mechanism for assessing observations, treatment, processes, experience, and/or outcomes of patient care

    – In other words, CQMs assess "the degree to which a provider competently and safely delivers clinical services that are appropriate for the patient in an optimal timeframe.

- **Registry:** organized system which uses observational study methods to collect uniform data (clinical and other) to evaluate specified outcomes for a population defined by a particular disease, condition, or exposure, and that serves 1 or more predetermined scientific, clinical, or policy purposes

- **Risk factor:** aspect of personal behavior/lifestyle, environmental exposure, or inborn/inherited characteristic that, on the basis of epidemiologic evidence, is known to be associated with health-related condition(s) considered important to prevent. (Last 2001)

- **Screening:** using tests or other methods of diagnosis to find out whether a person has a specific disease/condition before it causes any symptoms

    – For many diseases (e.g., cancers), starting treatment earlier leads to better results. The purpose of screening is to find the disease so that treatment can be started as early as possible. For example, a breast exam and mammogram are both screening tests used to find small breast cancers.

- **Social determinant:** proposed or established causal factor in the social environment which affects health outcomes (e.g., income, education, occupation, class, social support)

- **Target population:** entire service area or any subset, whether economic, geographic, or demographic, or individuals with certain health conditions

- **Upstream determinants:** features of the social environment, such as socioeconomic status and discrimination that influence individual behavior, disease, and health status

Practice Questions

1. A 59-year-old man with a history of type 2 diabetes is diagnosed with diabetic retinopathy and referred to ophthalmology for additional management. The patient's primary care physician is interested in reducing the number of patients in the practice who develop similar long-term complications from type 2 diabetes mellitus. Which one of the following is the most important next step?

    (A) Develop an intervention to monitor blood glucose levels for all patients in the practice

    (B) Utilize the patient registry to identify high-risk patients comprising the target population

    (C) Train staff in the clinic to identify early signs of retinopathy

    (D) Request to have an ophthalmologist perform fundoscopic exams on all patients in the practice

    (E) Place a sign in the office depicting the dangers of diabetes

Answer: B. One of the first steps in designing a population health management program is to define the target population and identify common risk factors or gaps in care. Ideally, this should be done prior to implementing any intervention, so that it is clear which patients have the greatest need for the intervention and what risk factor(s) the intervention should address.

*   Monitoring blood glucose for all patients, even those without diabetes or not at risk for diabetes, may not be a practical use of resources.

*   Training staff to identify retinopathy or having an ophthalmologist perform fundoscopic exams will identify patients who already have long-term complications, rather than adjusting behaviors to prevent complications.

*   A sign depicting the dangers of diabetes is not a proactive measure, does not optimally engage patients in self-care, and may only help those who are already in the clinic.

2. An 8-year-old boy is brought to the emergency department by his mother after he develops acute shortness of breath and wheezing. The boy appears anxious but is alert and responsive. He is afebrile and responds well to supplemental oxygen and initial respiratory treatment. He has a history of asthma and has presented with similar symptoms 4 times in the past 12 months. The mother smokes 1-2 packs of cigarettes per day while at home with her son. Which of the following addresses an upstream determinant of health amenable to population health management to improve the patient's long-term outcome?

    (A) Rapid use of nebulizer treatments in the emergency department

    (B) Administration of weight adjusted dose of steroid treatment

    (C) Asking the mom to purchase an inhaler to keep at the home

    (D) Parent education on second-hand smoking risk and enrollment in a smoking cessation program

    (E) Prophylactic antibiotics

Answer: D. Educating parents about the risks of second-hand smoke to children—especially one with a history of asthma—and offering parents enrollment in a smoking-cessation program may have a dramatic benefit to the health of the child and help prevent future asthma attacks. Use of nebulizers or steroids in the emergency department may be necessary to treat the acute episode of care; however, will not help prevent future attacks. The use of antibiotics without indications of bacterial infection (e.g. no fever) is not warranted.

Index

A

Abandonment of patients, 146

Abbreviations, "Do Not Use" list for, 188

Abortion
  adolescent pregnancy and, 105
  Roe vs Wade decision, 144
  state variations in laws about, 148

Absolute risk reduction, in observational studies, 120

Abuse, of substance. *See* Substance abuse; *individual substances*

Academic performance, measuring, 7

Accuracy, screening test performance, 112

Acting out, 6

Active euthanasia, 146

Active failures, in medical error, 181

Acute dystonia, 80

Acute movement syndromes, antipsychotics inducing, 80

Acute stress disorder (ASD), 29

Addictive disorders, 51–54
  gambling, 57
  overview of, 51–52

Addition, mutually exclusive events by, 129

Adjusted (standardized) rates, 97–98

Adjustment disorders, 49

Adolescents
  pregnancy in, 105
  sexual behavior in, 106

Advance directives, competency and, 145

Adverse effects
  of antidepressants, 81, 82
  of antipsychotics, 79–80
  of electroconvulsive therapy, 83
  of mood-stabilizers, 83, 84

Adverse events, 175
  contributing factors, 179–180
  prevention of, 186, 189, 195
  reporting of, 194
  second victim of, 183

Adverts, pharmaceutical, interpretation of, 160–161, 166–167

Affect, in mental status examination, 1

Age, disease rates positively correlated with, 98

Agnosia, 37

Agoraphobia, 27
  specific phobia vs., 28

Akathisia, 80

Alcohol
  effect on sleep, 69
  mild neurocognitive disorder and, 42

Alcohol abuse, 53

α error, in hypothesis testing, 136

Alternative hypothesis, 135

Amitriptyline, 82

Amnesia, dissociative, 45

Amnestic disorder(s), 42

Amniocentesis, in ID diagnosis, 9

Amphetamine abuse, 53

Anabolic steroids, abuse of, 53

Analysis of variance (ANOVA), 138, 140

Anchoring bias, diagnostic error and, 177

Anorexia nervosa, 59–60

ANOVA (analysis of variance), 138, 140

Antibiotic prophylaxis, selection and administration, 187

Anticholinergic effects
  from antidepressants, 81
  from antipsychotics, 79

Antidepressant medications. *See also individual medications*
  for adjustment disorders, 49
  clinical guidelines for, 81
  hybrid forms, 82
  monoamine oxidase inhibitors, 82
  for pseudodementia, 41
  selective serotonin reuptake inhibitors, 82
  tricyclic, 82
  untoward effects of, 81

Antipsychotic medications, 79–81. *See also individual medications*
  acute movement syndromes induced by, 80
  atypical, 79, 80–81
  general principles of, 79
  side effects of, 79–80
  typical, 79

Antisocial personality disorder, 65

Anxiety disorders
  acute stress disorder, 29
  in childhood, 13